# I Had to CHOOSE to Feel Better

# I Had to CHOOSE to Feel Better

**Asadah Kirkland**

Asadah Sense Consulting
Chicago, Illinois

## I Had to CHOOSE to Feel Better

Published by:
Asadah Sense Consulting
Chicago, Illinois
asadah@soulfulchicagobookfair.com

Asadah Kirkland, Publisher
Yvonne Rose/QualityPress.info, Book Packager

*I Had to CHOOSE to Feel Better* books are available at special discounts for bulk purchases, sales promotions, fundraising, or educational purposes. Call: 646-359-6605 for information and orders.

Disclaimer: This book is for informational purposes only and not meant to diagnose others or give medical advice. This book is a testament to Asadah Kirkland's healing process, and all observations involved during the healing discoveries.

Copyright © 2025 by Asadah Sense Consulting
ISBN: 978-0-9836205-1-8
Library of Congress Control Number: 2025913353

# Dedication

This book is dedicated to all those
who push through challenging experiences in life,
knowing that the main way to enhance
the future is to make it.

I Had to CHOOSE to Feel Better

# Acknowledgements

First and foremost, I must acknowledge my daughter Patience Kirkland, who saved my life. Had she not been home when I had my seizure/stroke in August 2024, I may not have been here to write this book. Mommy admires and appreciates you!

My mother, Juanita Vidal, gave me daily encouragement throughout this healing process. Talking to her was therapeutic for me and I am forever thankful.

Thank you to my brother, Andrew Kirkland, for coming to get me during those unexpected late nights in the hospital.

I appreciate my stepdad, Rawle Vidal, for always sending me wholistic health videos to learn from about the body and food.

Big shout outs to all of my Facebook family that helped me financially get through this hard time. It was Adrian Sky who asked my daughter, "Does your mom have a GoFundMe we can give to?" and it started an avalanche of support from so many people. I am so humbled and grateful to you all.

Thank you to Kadijah Solomon for being new to Chicago, yet for making dedicated trips to my home to deliver Body Comm sessions to me.

I also give thanks to my girl Nina S. who gave her time and energy to nurse me back to normalcy by doing my hair, performing Body Comm Sessions on me, going for walks, going grocery shopping, and introducing me to drinking celery juice every morning to lower my blood pressure. She came out of nowhere and just cared for me when I really needed it.

When it comes to helping me restore balance in my body, The Natural Health Improvement Center was second to none! They made sure I maintained nutritionally balanced progress throughout my entire healing period...and it's still going.

I must acknowledge Penney Jack, Joy Sigur, Ernest Abdullah, Lisa Hardaway and Senabella Gill for my needed trips to get sustenance, when going to the store by myself was not yet possible. Thank you so much for caring for me.

And lastly, thank you to Asabi Carrol for her daily check-ins and nutritional advice the whole way through my healing journey.

# Contents

# Look It Up

There is a glossary in the back of this book. Sometimes we believe we know certain words, but the context of how they're being used is different from the definition we know. If you come across a word you are not sure of…LOOK IT UP! We don't want you not completing the book because you ran up against a word you don't know.

WHEREVER YOU SEE AN "I" PUT A "YOU" IF IT FITS.

This is an account of my life post-second stroke and first-time seizure. While the content of this book is specific to me, feel free to substitute the word "you" wherever you see me say the word "I" if it applies to you. We may have similar experiences regarding how we've dealt with ourselves. I simply mustered up the courage to put it in a book so we can all learn together and make life better for ourselves.

# Introduction

Much of what determines whether I healed or not had to do with my choice to think like a VICTIM or think like a VICTOR. Victim mode usually meant depending on sources outside of myself for comfort. Victor mode meant I was going to create a solution at all costs. This book is about my choosing to win and how I did it.

I do not remember a time in my life when I paid this much attention to my body and how it works. These days, I am aware of every little feeling in every inch of my body. Is it paranoia? Nope. It's a health study of myself. I've gone through most of my years being negligent…and I thought I was on the healthy spectrum. Turns out, I needed to educate myself more about what exactly has been happening on the inside of me. The part of me I can't see is more important than ever now. I wrote this book so that the reader considers their own health journey and important steps to take to make it a good one.

This book was written for the person who keeps putting their better health on the back burner. It's written for those of us who keep making excuses for why we eat things that we know we should NOT eat. Being disciplined in diet does not always come easy. It first takes a decision, and then it takes work. Sometimes it takes sacrifice and not getting our way. Other times, it takes ignoring the things we KNOW will hurt us. Some of the things we ingest make us lethargic, some things make us drunk, some things make us feel sick, and some things take a little time, but cause us to deteriorate. This book is about eliminating discomfort and replacing it with calm. This book talks about how I got rid of the mystery of my body and its functioning and replaced it with certainty. This book is about seeing how one can make positive changes in his/her body towards a win. This book encourages research about the things that will help build you.

Do you even know anyone who is winning health-wise... physically...mentally...emotionally? The balance between them all is necessary. It's challenging to aim for something you've never really seen. My advice is to simply make your own attempt to feel optimal. People often complain about aches and pains and body problems, but how often do we come across people who do the opposite? This book is about articulating the good things going on in our bodies. I've become a better resource to others on how to take good care of oneself.

This book is NOT for people who give up. This book is not for the immature person who just doesn't give a crap and feels that they are going to die anyway. This book is not for people with no purpose in life. This book is for those who KNOW there is a reason they are on this planet. This book is for the people who love themselves enough to improve themselves. I wrote this book after realizing that the world does not benefit from my being inadequate, mediocre, or average. I fully realize that there is a BEST person I can be, and only I can make the decision to do the things that help me be that. I feel like perfection is a great aim. The word wouldn't exist if it wasn't real. It's just relevant to each person's actuality of themselves. Each person has their own perfect. Not reaching it is a choice, yet aiming for it is admirable.

Take this book and share its power! Use my example as a guide to follow if FEELING BETTER is something you want to experience. No one wants aches, pains, itching, nausea, dizziness, and such. This book is about addressing the ultimate you that you want to be. If we all aim to feel our best, I believe that will lead to us acting our best, which should then lead to creating our best…decisions, relationships, and conditions. So, enjoy my healing journey. This book was written to set an example and create some dialogue about how we can improve ourselves for the time we have on this planet. Feel better with me! Game start!

# SPIRIT

## TESTIMONY

More than anything, this book is a testimony. I had a big choice to make, and that choice was to either be a victim or a victor after my health incident in August 2024. Having both a stroke and a seizure was no joke for me. When you get hurt or something happens to you that is damaging to your mind, body, and spirit, you have to figure out a way to overcome that trauma. For me, overcoming that trauma was a choice. I could have sat and waited for others to help me, but I had to decide to improve myself at some point. That is what this book is about. It is my testimony and the way I handled being hurt, getting through it, and recuperating toward better health.

This book even looks at my acknowledgment of the pain I put myself through, which can be the hardest pain to overstand and move past. Prayer is good, but choosing to do better and being disciplined is needed to strengthen the prayers. This road of healing is not an easy road by any stretch of the imagination. This time is full of challenges and fear, and sometimes even confusion. The key has become to push past those things, because I know I have a purpose in life that is greater than any of those things. My conversations with God give me the strength I know it takes to reach higher. I am clear that it takes a force greater than just myself to come through it all. It gets to the point where I must see that communicating with God IS communicating with myself. I reflect the Most High. That power IS my power. And seeing myself through that lens…that grand…has been the force needed to create the future. The hurt is in the past. It's the FUTURE that holds all the possibilities I have yet to create.

This book is a place for you to walk through with me, see what I did, and then help make choices to do what you must do to become your best self. At the point of writing this book, I am not even my best self yet, but I am definitely on the road to a great recovery. There's a lot of deducing and processes of elimination on how to best take care of myself. I don't just take the word of sources outside of me. I listen to God FIRST and then let the rest of the world chime in at my discretion. I look forward to the life that I know I've worked for, and I am leaving behind the world where I don't do my best. Thank you for joining this journey, and let's be powerful together. Choose it!

## IT'S A SPIRITUAL THANG

There is a force in each of our lives that can't be denied. It's not about what you believe in. It's what you FEEL. It governs how you interact with the environment around you. It's made up of things you can't see, yet you know exist. It's the stuff that deja'vu is made of. It comes from the same place as when you think of someone, and they surprisingly appear. It's when it's 3:30 am and the message comes through crystal clear…and you better get up and write it down.

Some of you have hovered over your body and watched yourself sleep. Those dreams seem so real. Yeah, it's the things you KNOW but can't physically touch. All these manifestations and more happen in the spiritual realm. It's where our power lies. Unfortunately, we don't trust this realm all the time. We often wait until we reach times of adversity and experience "awakenings" of some sort. The truth of the matter is that our abilities have always been with us. In times past, we were in tune with these abilities on another level. God wasn't far away. I believe we've lessened our communication with God over the centuries and allowed sources outside of ourselves to guide us.

Each of us is a vessel with a specific calling and contribution to make while we're here on this earth. That calling is evident in a human being, even after just being on this plane for two years. All we have to do is watch and listen. Let intuition lead instead of having to see things with your eyeballs all the time. Our whole individual journey is a calling for each of us individually to make an impact. Find what that is and get to it! Let KNOWING guide you. If you KNOW something isn't good for you, don't do it! If you KNOW something feels good and right, DO IT! God got you! The Creator just wants to see if we've got ourselves.

That's right. Make the decision to master yourself and BE the you that intends to be a light to the world. If you keep your journey spiritual, all you're doing is doing you…you ARE a spirit in a human body, remember. Be the value you were sent here to be. Value your specific self. Enjoy you, and the Creator will appear to enact the you She/He sent you here for all along. Your time is precious…now go act like it and create your magic!

# SUNLIGHT

If you know anything about me, it's that I take pictures and videos of the sunrise every morning I can. I live right on Lake Michigan, here in Chicago, and I have no…I repeat…no man-made obstruction of the sun rising. I've often called the Sun "Sunita." It's a play on my mom's name, "Juanita." Oftentimes, I cannot believe I don't see other faces in all of the windows of my building, watching the same scene I see as the Sun rises. We all know that it's the Earth revolving that lends the appearance of the Sun rising off the horizon, yet that's not what matters.

No matter how you choose to look at it, it's all a spiritual, celestial phenomena of the Most High. I've become somewhat of a scientist and have observed that if the clock gives a time for the sunrise, you have to be ready to view it two minutes before that time if you want to see the start of the rising process. You'll miss it if you aren't ready two minutes before.

This is my quiet time of the day. I get to witness colors and shapes of God that you usually can only capture on television or in movies. I've watched the sky turn into purples and pinks before the Sun actually emerges, and I've witnessed the clouds break the Sun in half as she rises to higher heights of the day. I am grateful for my sunrise moments. The beauty is that those moments can exist for all of us. It's simply about the choice to be in a place where you can capture the same scene for yourself in your part of the world. And it's free to see. I often parallel the rise of the Sun to my own persistence and willingness to rise in my own life. The clouds represent life's obstacles, yet I always acknowledge the interaction of them and the Sun and the beauty that is created regardless of how the Sun moves through them. And on cloudy days when the view of the Sun is fully obstructed, I keep in mind that THERE WOULD BE NO DAYLIGHT without the Sun's presence. The correlation to me? Shine my light no matter what…it makes a difference to someone all the time, even when I am not aware of my impact.

Take time to enjoy the Sun. Beyond being beautiful, it gives us much-needed Vitamin D and is available to supply the world with energy.

## GET READY FOR THE DOWNLOADS

My decisions are made from listening to a source that's connected to my spiritual awareness. I mentioned it earlier, yet it's that time of the morning when your ideas for the day are floating all over the place in your dream state. As a matter of fact, sometimes it's hard to tell if you are asleep or not. I know one thing, though. The message to get up and write down what you're thinking is always front and center. I call these moments DOWNLOADS. It is my belief that God tells me what to do and how to do it when I get those downloads. In my experience, if I don't jot it down, I lose the details of the assignment. I do not go back and forth with these downloads. Whatever comes through, I get to work on the idea immediately.

Every big idea I've embarked on came through a download. I don't use my own man-made ideas and opinions to compare what I receive in a download. I confront those God-given assignments with intention and specificity. In my mind, the information is given with just the right stuff that helps me organize my thoughts and set the necessary parameters. There's nothing to question when I receive those downloads. I'm the vessel the Most High uses to implement those exact ideas. Even if the task seems large, I know I can achieve it because of how it was delivered to me. Have you ever received a download as described above? If so, what was it?

_____

_____

_____

I feel like the downloads are part of the purpose for why we exist. The downloads usually align with the impact we're supposed to make in this world. Don't fear the work! If the assignment came in a download, God got your back!

## YOUR VOICE VS GOD'S VOICE

Oh yeah...you will hear voices during a time of healing BIG TIME! No, I'm not talking about some type of psycho trip. There will be what's called intuition, or your first mind. It's what you KNOW in your gut. That's God communicating. Too often, we argue back and forth with that voice. We rationalize and question what we FEEL. That's the human being in us talking. One might ask, "How can you tell the difference?" In my opinion, you can tell the human thought from the innate gut thought because it's usually based on some type of fear or doubt that makes you question your intuition. I've found that when I make decisions from that KNOWING space, everything works out best. Plan A's usually come from that KNOWING space and excitement. Then here comes plan B…full of maybes, doubts, and fear of the easiness of Plan A.

Here's an idea! How about seeing that God talking through you IS you! Once the guidance comes into your mind, IT'S YOU! Listening to that KNOWING God space is a choice you can make. It's made of stuff that doesn't come written on paper until you put it there. Everything around you came from that imaginative space. Thank goodness for people who know how to take their ideas and bring them to fruition. And we can be thankful for their courage to do so. This book was written to show how I chose to follow that God- KNOWING space when taking care of myself. I had to think beyond faith and act out of KNOWING. Faith looks outside of oneself for answers. KNOWING takes instruction from God, via the person in the mirror. We are used to taking guidance from others outside of ourselves, so what I'm saying takes practice. Practice following what you KNOW. I got great results when I did and used the assistance of others to add to my God-planned program.

# MIND

## I WASN'T RAISED LIKE THAT

How could I let something that severe occur? When I thought about it, no one in my upbringing was health-conscious. No one spoke of nutrients and what foods were needed to keep the body functioning well. It just wasn't a topic of discussion. Weight loss and diets were discussed at times. There was no knowledge being shared about eating foods that were helpful to us, though. This goes for most Black communities throughout the US. Kool-Aid and quarter waters were the beverages of choice. Thereafter came the sodas, and Mountain Dew was my personal favorite. There was no care in the world about how much sugar was in those bottles, let alone what was happening on the inside of the body because of them.

"Soul Food," huh? Diabetes and High Blood Pressure perhaps came from such cooking. Of course, the TASTE was divine, yet contributing to the quality of one's SOUL it did not. This is not to make us wrong for preparing food the way we do. We should simply begin to take inventory of the foods we ingest, and the results created when eating them. Being from NYC, we didn't have a big emphasis on eating soul food. We grew up getting fast food galore. Mom cooked, but I remember getting chicken wings and French fries drenched in ketchup from the Chinese restaurant. And we had to go through a bar to get to the restaurant, as little kids, no less. No one stopped us either. That five-dollar meal was ssoooo satisfying and full of oils and salt. I know it did not make a good contribution to our bodies. But who cares when you're young, right? I'm writing this book because we must start caring. Killing ourselves slowly affects the QUALITY of the life we live and the decisions we make.

I had to come to grips with my over-reliance on processed foods: I had dietary habits that included a high intake of processed foods, like vegetarian meats specifically. I had to take a look at how my food was packaged, and if it came in a box, I probably should stay away from it. Fresh, whole foods that had very little ingredient content had to become my priority. Whatever I chose had to be the main or ONLY ingredient in the item of my choosing.

## VULNERABILITY

The word vulnerability has about four or five definitions. The one I want to use here is: *willingness to show emotion or to allow one's weaknesses to be seen or known.* I can honestly say that I was not used to showing vulnerability prior to my seizure and stroke in August 2024. Going into the hospital with a sugar level over 500mg/dl, high cholesterol, high blood pressure, and the like, made the body physically weak.

Then here came that MENTAL weakness trotting close behind. This is where I had to make decisions to live or die. There was no hiding at that point. Not only was weakness all over the place for everyone to see, but there were also moments when I wanted hand-holding and help and forces outside of myself to make me strong. *Guess what?* There was nothing outside of me to make me strong without the will to BE strong myself.

Oh boy, was it easy to succumb to feelings that circled around crying and giving up. Yet, my purposes were more powerful. Purpose kept me afloat. It's how this book even got here. I want to live well throughout my daughter's life and influence her decisions with my example. She has seen me vulnerable more than anyone during this time. My choice is to drown those images of vulnerability with new images of future-building and perseverance.

While I've always been used to being strong and wise, I do embrace this small moment in time of vulnerability. At least I know I can be it. I just choose NOT to be it. I prefer to show emotion that inspires people to do better. I enjoy leading by example. I've learned that folks are not comfortable when strong people need holding up. There's not a lot of physical support up here in "Leaderville." This is where INNER strength came in. Choosing to feel better meant pushing through all challenges. Worry presented itself at every corner, yet I had to replace worry with facts and practice. That's what this book demonstrates. This book shares much of what I learned and applied. Now that I've shown my weaknesses, it's time for me to get over them. Words of wisdom…GET YOUR PURPOSES IN ORDER! My purposes always direct me toward the future. If I don't like what I see, then I'd better create another actuality.

The main point is for me not to get STUCK in vulnerable. Being resilient is a plus! Being strong is a plus! I'm not here to ignore being vulnerable, yet I prefer CAUSING things to happen instead of being the EFFECT of them happening.

## TO FEEL BETTER

Sometimes I felt so bad that it was challenging to even imagine feeling good. I think it's easy to stay in the "feeling bad" space, because it usually comes with pity . Folks say they don't like being pitied, but I believe they do. It's the stuff sympathy and being called a poor baby are made of. I want you to take some time to actually imagine what having no pain and problems feels like. Think of days when you really enjoyed yourself and filled your world with laughter. Remember a time when you were creating something and got satisfaction from your laser focus. Think about waking up with plans and getting up ready to achieve them. I found that to obtain my "feeling better," I had to take inventory of what those things are that put me in a state of feeling and acting better.

To FEEL better, I had to:

- Listen to the downloads from the Creator.
- Make a shift in my eating habits.
- Take full responsibility for myself, my actions, and physical condition
- Create a clear purpose as to why living was a better option than dying.

- Get Body Comm sessions.

- Drink celery juice every morning.

- Keep the body moving.

- Research and learn the exact foods and vitamins my body called for that could assist me in my healing process.

- Eliminate parasites from my body.

- Dance.

- Walk & exercise.

- Listen to HERTZ-specific frequencies of music.

- Breathe in negative ions from moving water outside my window.

- Go to the Energy Enhancement Center.

- Visit with my own Nutritionist.

- Learn to breathe to bring my Blood Pressure down naturally.

- Research foods and vitamins to lower my cholesterol.

- Get A1C in normal range.

- Control blood pressure and keep it in normal range.

- Be disciplined and not allow myself to eat anything that didn't bring me good health.

- Watch Little House on the Prairie.

To feel better, I had to begin a TRUE assessment of what I put in my mouth as food and what effect it was having on my body. I had to choose to decide what was normal for me to eat. It's not about restrictions and looking at what I could no longer eat. It became more about how I wanted to FEEL and what abilities I wanted to maintain and enhance.

I had to eliminate fear. I don't know about you, but fear is not associated with any emotion I want to experience. Fear is steeped in doubt. Fear usually comes from something being unknown. Better yet, I feel what we fear is simply what we're not willing to look at. What I've found is that as soon as I made the choice to look at that thing (whatever was ailing me), it lessened its power. I could address it and overcome it if necessary. Not knowing what is happening in and to my body was scary to me. The minute I confronted the unwanted feelings and researched what I could do to gain control, the scariness ceased. Little by little, I created a better me. I applied what I learned and made better disciplined decisions about taking care of myself. Some things were new to me, yet I knew they were better for me than what I DIDN'T use to do.

## LYING TO MYSELF

So, what's the problem with lying to ourselves? Lying to ourselves is something many of us experience, whether it's small self-deceptions or larger, more impactful ones. These lies can serve to protect ourselves from uncomfortable truths, avoid facing fears or failures, or maintain an IMAGE of control and stability.

One of the main things I had to face before any healing could take place was how much I had been lying to myself. *Why?* Because I got wrapped up in BELIEVING the base of how I thought and what I did. The major lie for me was that I didn't eat meat, I never got high, never smoked, and never drank, so I was GOOD as far as health was concerned. Keeping all of that at the forefront of my mind, I ignored signs of other things I allowed to enter my body that were CLEARLY not making me feel better. Just because they didn't make me feel bad at the time, I made it seem like they had invisible effects on me...or no effect on me at all. The lie became me not being truthful about what I allowed myself to ingest. I wasn't HIDING that I ate some pizza, had some chips, or ate something else that caused an adverse effect, I just didn't promote it.

The best way to deal with this sneaky aspect of myself was to simply CONFRONT the truth. Taking inventory of everything that enters my digestive system and observing the effects they have on how I feel has become a lifestyle for me now. Sometimes I want to chew gum so badly, but I just won't do it. I cannot justify what's being released into my saliva, nor can I link it to anything good that will happen to my body after I ingest it. I know it says "sugar-free" on the wrapper, but that's not all it says. To ignore all the other chemicals listed on the label because I may not overstand the impact those ingredients have on me is not a good choice for me to make. When I look at the amount of gum I used to chew daily...multiply all of those chemicals going in my body on a daily basis...there's no telling if any of that contributed to my final illness. The main illness was indeed my making, like the unwanted chemicals had zero effects on me. This was another lie to tell myself, to take away my responsibility to Asadah. If I don't take care of me, who will?

## MY NEGLIGENCE AFFECTED OTHERS

When seeing folks do damaging things to themselves like smoking or drinking, I've heard people say things like, "You gonna die anyway." Now, while I've never had that viewpoint and never said anything like that, I certainly IGNORED things I did that were harmful to me. Harming myself meant eating bread that I loved or ingesting chips and cookies. Yeah, I always felt good about not eating meat for decades, but I acted as if I didn't know starch turned to sugar. I knew my body was not working properly enough to handle that sugary situation that starches make, but I ate what I wanted anyway. One of the huge problems with not taking care of oneself is not considering how our decisions affect others.

For me, I hate that my daughter had to experience my illness at such a young age. When I had my first stroke in 2009, I did not let her come see me in the hospital…and I was there for approximately 3 months! When I got out of the hospital back then, my daughter had to watch me violently vomiting every day and staying in bed until I was able to walk on my own again. Thereafter, she had to watch me walk, assisted by a cane. Fast forward to my most recent stroke and seizure, my daughter literally had to do compressions on me to revive me. I hate that she has that record of me in her mind, stored in her memory banks. My being on the bathroom floor unconscious, bleeding, and near death came from my decision to ingest so much starch that it sent my sugar level to over 500mg/dl. And I knew better.

My daily sugar level was always between 250mg/dl -350mg/gl on average. A stroke was always moments away, and I kept ignoring that reality. I figured that if I felt okay, then there should not have been much to worry about. Very wrong, Asadah. My daughter is a laid-back young woman and never lets on to how much stress this incident has caused her. Not only did she save my life, but she also administered my insulin daily, talked to nurses in my stead, cooked my meals…all before she was even 21 years of age. One should mature, yes. Yet one should not be forced into any kind of traumatic maturation. My daughter had to take on adult responsibilities without preparation and potentially has mental scarring because of it.

Moral of the story…before we engage in situations that put us in harm's way, think about the people around us who are going to have your choice trickle over into their lives…causing more turmoil. Every choice we make has a ripple effect on another person's life. Making a positive choice will ripple out, too. As I continue to heal and send my daughter good reports about my improved health, I keep in mind the comfort and confidence I want her to have for her mother. I do not want her to lead a young life having to take care of her grown a%# mother.

## MY OWN BEST ADVOCATE

A hard lesson to learn during my healing process was to take MYSELF as an authority on ME. This is not about not listening to doctors. It became about deciding on whom I'd pay most attention to regarding my own body. I looked to ME for help. If I got myself into that mess, it meant I could get myself out of it, too. It's easy to ask a doctor what's wrong with you physically. We usually feel secure because they went to school to learn about the body and how it works…so we believe. It turns out that the study of medicines seems to get highlighted by doctors, yet the study of foods to help heal one naturally is not studied by the majority of them.

Don't get me wrong, I was the first one to be thankful for the medical help I received when I had my seizure/stroke incident. Nonetheless, it became extremely important to monitor myself and help make decisions that suited me best, according to my comfort and goal to operate as my best me. It's important to know that Help Is Not Outside of You. Taking too much chemical medicine was NOT a place I wanted to be in. I watched my grandmother die that way. Finding out the natural equivalent to those chemicals is where I put my focus. It required daily research by me to find what I needed to increase in my diet. I weaned myself off the various medicines the doctors gave me and let them know when and why I did. I had discussions with them about my changes. Even if they didn't fully articulate support for my choices, I had to know what was working for me through observation.

I took their blood tests, yet I also maintained my visits to my Nutritionist. Taking supplements based on what I wanted to achieve for myself is how I healed naturally. Working with the Nutritionist took the guesswork out of my healing. I felt more assured knowing that when I left the Nutritionist. The supplements I took home were all food-based and not chemicals made in a laboratory. Thank you, Natural Health Improvement Center!

## FEELING ALONE

I don't remember feeling as lonely as I felt during the healing process of this last traumatic experience. Don't get me wrong. I had a tremendous outpouring of financial support from friends on social media, fellow NU alums, fellow Scientologists, and the like. And there are no words for the level of support I got from my own daughter, Patience! Patience stepped up to the plate and literally kept me living. Once they sent me home from the hospital, my daughter did everything from cooking my meals to administering insulin needles every morning.

I'll always feel that I wore her out, yet she didn't complain. I could see the sadness and tiredness in her eyes, though. Once it was time for her to go back to work and college, I knew I'd pretty much have to fend for myself. Much of that time was extremely lonely.

Now there's loneliness and there's solitude. Solitude is being by oneself and feeling good or relieved because of it. Feeling alone is a whooooole other animal. When you feel alone, it's like your mind starts playing tricks on you. When you're by yourself, fear can rear its ugly head, and you can start imagining all kinds of negative ideas. *So, how should you combat that feeling?* All I can tell you is what I did.

For some, prayer comes in this space of feeling alone. I think it's important not to beg God for what you want, though. The answer to your healing and sanity still sits in YOU...remember that. During prayer, I'd ask for clarity about your situation. I'd ask for the removal of fear and the addition of courage. Now, I told you I'd tell you what I chose to do. I know I did a whole lot of napping during these lonely times. Napping helped me NOT confront the fact that I was alone, and the body heals while you sleep, too. But you can't nap all the time.

I began to collect songs and add them to one long streaming album. I chose songs that made me smile when they played...nostalgic songs like "Knocks Me Off My Feet" by Stevie Wonder, "Destiny" by the Jacksons, "Summertime Madness" by Kool and the Gang, or "Sparrow" by Marvin Gaye. Before I knew it, I was playing a game of remembering songs that used to mean a lot to me. I even made an album called "Blue-eyed Soul Brothers," and added songs like "Madge" by Steven Bishop, "Roxanne" by the Police, or "Screen Kiss" by Thomas Dolby. All these songs helped me reflect on good times and helped me sing again. Before I knew it, I chose to dance for social media sometimes. The key was to add activities to my new, post-incidence lifestyle that made me feel good, even doing them by myself.

When I was alone, I'd want to feel like a victim at times. I just wanted a person to be there that I could lay my head on. Sometimes I just wanted to have someone to talk to or cry to. But being the positive person I am, I had to turn my frown upside down and figure out the reason I was alone. One thing I know for sure is that being alone forced me to take full responsibility for healing myself. If I had a home attendant helping me or something, I would have stayed in bed being served and not training myself to cook for myself and move around.

Today I am thankful for my alone time. I know I became a better listener to God, as well as to my body. Listening to my body became of the utmost importance. I would listen and then research what to do to improve anything that wasn't normal to me. I took a ton of new normals to live by. I also took on an enhanced appreciation for reaching out to people. If someone came to mind, I started calling them instead of letting the thought of them just pass away in the wind. There were days when I wondered, "Where are all my friends? Why aren't more people reaching out to me?" That's when I had to ask myself, "How much did you reach out to check up on people before your incident, Asadah?"

I like my newfound "Just checkin' up on ya" calls. I rekindled friendships of old and made decisions to keep new friendships alive because they fostered new experiences and new conversations about new topics. I also learned that I will only experience the things I CHOOSE to create.

Making sure I had projects to work on and deadlines for them helped me rehabilitate my use of alone time as well. From filling out grant applications to writing this book, I kept myself busy with meaningful work. That meant my PURPOSE had to be intact. So, while you're alive enough to be alone, figure out the PURPOSE of your being alone. There's probably a lesson there somewhere...maybe a few lessons for that matter. As soon as you identify them, start acting on them. That alone time will turn out to be quiet time for creating if you let it.

## BEING AWARE

Have you ever heard, "What you don't know won't hurt you." That is a bold-faced lie if I've ever heard one. Not being aware of ANY circumstance can only lead you to being a victim of sorts. Being aware puts one in a position to be able to CAUSE whatever you desire in any circumstance. It was a major problem that I wasn't aware that starch turned to sugar. As a result, I became a victim of the bad circumstance of eating too much food that was killing me. Once I became aware of the foods that were destroying me, it was time to take responsibility for taking in foods that would reverse the damage.

Now, my awareness of what my body does and needs is bananas! And I STILL have a lot more to learn and apply! I've taken an awareness of my body's irregularities and turned them into new, applied processes for a better, healthier life for myself. Unfortunately, I got a harsh reality and awareness of what an awful health situation feels like. And from it, I was able to compare and gain an awareness of the types of tools I needed to fix this old gal's body. Once you know, you KNOW. Once you know, you can take responsibility for yourself and how you feel. From then you'll have better control of your health-related outcomes. What are you AWARE of regarding your body?

_____

_____

_____

_____

## DO YOU WANT TO DIE?

Now wait a minute! Let's be clear. There's nothing in this book or in my entire universe that is suicidal. If there are two things all humans are going to do, it's live and die. That's right, we are all going to expire. We know it's coming. But just because we know it's coming doesn't mean we have to live a life bringing it on earlier than it needs to be here. Time and time again, I see people doing things to their bodies, not thinking about the effects they're creating. Folks smoke cigarettes, drink liquor, use drugs, and such. And guess what I hear waaay too many people say? "Well, we're gonna die anyway." This just happens to be what many people say when they are doing something they know is damaging to their body, but they don't want to take responsibility for it. People say this as an excuse or justification for doing something they

KNOW is not good for their well-being. Let them start dying! Then you see a change of heart.

I've seen chain smokers turn into wheatgrass drinkers, trying to save their own lives. By that time, it's usually too late, though. Unfortunately, it's usually too late to start repairing the body. And while I personally have never said this, I have absolutely ignored eating things I knew were bad for my health. No more denial for me, I tell you!

I'm at the point in my life now where I am preventing any further damage. Having two strokes and a seizure was enough to make me value my life the way I should. I know for a fact that I have never taken this much care of myself in all of my 54 years of life. One of my main weapons is to think about how I DON'T want to feel. We can all do that, right? We know what pain and suffering can feel like and allow ourselves to revisit those feelings all too often.

Now that I feel what GOOD HEALTH feels like, I'm not willing to experience the badness anymore. The problem is that people don't have a good reference point for what good health FEELS like. We watch it on television, on others, but that's them and not us. Take a minute and think about what you'd REALLY like to feel like. Describe it on the lines below:

_____

_____

_____

Now, look at what you wrote down and research what foods you need to eat to help that state. Then look at the vitamins and minerals you need to bring about that state. Then look up the movements you need to do to contribute to that state. Pretty soon, you'll see a lifestyle formed from the new practices and habits you have. And at that point, you'll be able to tell the difference between NOT feeling good and FEELING REAL GOOD!

## GAME PLAYING

We always played games in my house growing up. We played Chutes and Ladders, Candyland, Monopoly, Pokeno, Atari, Nintendo, and countless other games. As an adult, I indulge in phone video games daily…at all hours of my 24 hrs. Yet, I'm not here to talk about these types of games. What I've found is that I've approached life as a game for quite some time. What I had to identify in recent times is "What life game am I playing right now?" Getting hurt doesn't put you in a winning frame of mind. And I love winning!

Well, when an athlete gets injured, can he still play his game? He or she usually cannot. So, imagine how I felt having a seizure and a stroke! Since then, I don't dance as much, and I am limited when it comes to social activities I can attend. What?! Limits?! I hate them! The reality I had to face is that I took on a new type of game once I got injured. That game involves me not being as strong and looking outside of myself to move on the board. Decision time! *Is this a game I'm willing to play?* I am used to creating games and then playing them to win! Going on, taking insulin and high blood pressure medicine every day is NOT the life game I want to play. The game I want to play involves freedom to move without limits. The new game I want to play involves me operating as a strong, healthy being that inspires others to do the same. My girl, Angela, made it so clear to me in one of our conversations about my current health situation and said, "This life of medicine and worry is a losing game." Ooooweee, did that have the impact I needed it to have!

When I looked at my life as a game, in a new unit of time, I began to look at playing this health game the way I know I can. Now came the strategy. Now came looking at the life I WANT and not the life I don't want. Now came looking at who I want on my team and thinking like a victor and not a victim. The mind games of failure and weakness had to be outrun by activities of achievement. Looking at life as a game shifted my power button. I found myself feeling powerless and chose to change my mode to power-filled.

This may sound easier said than done, but I say…JUST GET ER' DONE! Figure out your purpose and play the game towards your goal. My current game is BIGGER than becoming healthy. Becoming healthy is a smaller game WITHIN the game of creating great things for others. Whatever I choose, I must add playfulness and insouciance to getting the end result. Seriousness and sadness ain't gonna cut it. This book has become part of my game playing toward a win and confronting all the parts of life that help me get there.

I Had to CHOOSE to Feel Better

# BODY

# FEELING "JACKED UP"

Okay, so what had happened was…

Let's take it back to 2008. I was diagnosed with new-onset Diabetes, with a sugar level of 470 mg/dl. One's sugar should be no higher than 125 mg/dl, mind you. I lived in NYC, and my daily diet consisted of carbs galore. I know there are people out there saying that having Diabetes has nothing to do with eating a lot of carbs, but I beg to differ. The truth of MY matter is that those starch-based foods did nothing good to my body (we'll talk more about that later). I was eating Chinese food daily. I was eating burritos with tons of vegetables…mega rice too, and whatever I wanted. Now, one would consider my food to be pretty clean because it was all "fresh." The reality, though, was that I was overworking my body by giving it foods it couldn't properly digest, and it showed. That 470 mg/dl of my blood level and undue NYC stress led me right into a stroke. That was my first stroke.

In late July 2024, my second stroke was accompanied by a seizure. I knew my eating habits were crusin' for a brusin.' I had great salads for lunch, but boy was I adding fries, chips, and cookies to my daily menu. I was drinking a flavored water that was said to have 1gm of sugar, every single day, right along with several sticks of gum to boot. I logged my sugar levels daily and sported numbers like 250 mg/dl – 350 mg/dl on a regular basis. On the day of my most recent and last stroke incident, I should have known I was pushing things to the limit. I had my regular super salad for lunch. I decided towards the end of it that I wanted some fries to finish things off. When I got home, my daughter had some soft, delicious, dairy-free cookies that I chose to add to the day's lot. I may have eaten almost half the pack if not more.

So here came how this got translated into a major physical problem. I was typing on my computer later that evening, and my left hand began to shake as if I had Parkinson's Disease. My fingertips were touching, and it was as if my hand was aiming for the screen like it was a touchscreen computer. The problem was not just the shaking, though. The bigger problem was that my mind could not control the hand's movement. I could not put my fingers back down onto the computer keys. Then my head began to shake, going repeatedly from left to right. I had to grab my left arm with my right hand to stop it from shaking. My solution to this was lying down. Sleep can be such an overutilized way to not confronting things.

Soon after I went to sleep, in the middle of the night, I got up for a bathroom break. Everything seemed ok…until it wasn't. Before I got off the seat of the toilet, my hand started to shake from left to right again…this time a little stronger. My head started to do as before, but this time more pronounced. My brain could not control either of the movements, and before I knew it, my shaking left arm began to uncontrollably twist backward. That's when I screamed my daughter's name, and it was lights out from there. I had no sense of the time that had lapsed. All I could see above me was my nervous daughter saying, "Please, mommy, come on mommy…" yet I did not know what she was talking about. A few minutes later, I saw a fireman above me, too. I was lying on the floor of the bathroom. I had a black eye, my mouth was bloody, and as I slowly awoke from unconsciousness, the firefighters stood me up and I was on my way to the hospital.

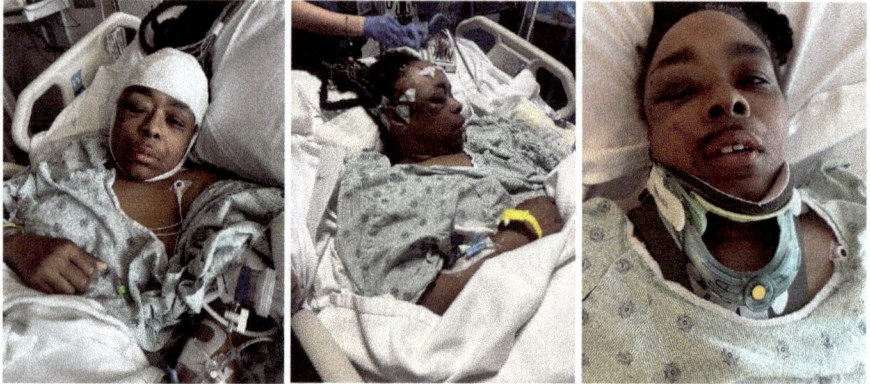

They put a neck brace on me and rushed me to the University of Chicago's hospital. From what my daughter tells me, she had to revive me. Dang, did I die a little bit? All I know is that the shaking happened once again while in the hospital, and they quelled it. My daughter told me that they stuck a tube down my throat, but I have no recollection of that. This was all a horrible scene. I hate that my daughter had to go through that. What a terrible price to pay for lacking discipline. I live differently now. This new life is designed to never let anything this atrocious happen again.

## LISTENING TO MY BODY TALK

If there is one thing I've truly learned during my healing process, it's listening to my body and then giving it what it needs to operate well. I have never in my life taken care of myself on this level. As I stated earlier, being a vegan had been the only commitment I made to taking care of myself. And yes, not eating flesh in a society that is gluttonous about eating dead bodies is commendable. When I stopped eating meat in 1990, I experienced shorter menstrual cycles and eliminated cramps. I knew then that I had made the correct decision to stop eating meat. I had a boyfriend at the time who cooked vegan food and introduced me to the lifestyle. Big ups Ngoni Simba! While this new way of eating contributed to sharper thinking, too, it did not address all the other foods out there that would impact my body negatively later in life.

My second stroke and first seizure set a different tone for me when it comes to how I deal with and have been learning about my body. The number one difference between this time and having a stroke the first time around was having to tend to myself, without a lot of physical help. My daughter helped with my meals and functioning until it was time for her to go back to school and work. I had applied for a home attendant, yet their telling me that they'd call me back for an appointment in a month meant that I had to fend for myself in the meantime. This meant that it was just me and God on this healing journey. When I think about it…CLEARLY THAT WAS THE BEST CHOICE ANY OLE WAY!

I became aware of every little sound and every feeling of discomfort everywhere in my body. Many times, I did not know what the feelings or sounds were but thank goodness for the internet. I became a researching bandit! There was a whistling in my ear that I would only hear when I laid down. It sounded like it was wheezing. It was not from my respiratory system, though. All I knew is that I did not like knowing what caused it. I had other pressing issues to tend to and just chose to strengthen my body all around, and before I knew it, the sound never came back.

So, let's talk about those other pressing issues, or should I say, how my body talked to me. Once, there was a vibration in my foot. It felt like when your phone vibrates when it's ringing, and it's sitting on your body. I timed it and saw that the vibrations were happening in my right foot every 10 seconds. I'm thankful that it was not pain, but I just knew it wasn't normal. Research came to the rescue! I looked up "vibration in foot." Turns out I was massively vitamin B12 deficient! Who knew?! My homegirl Asabi, tried to tell me that I needed B12 earlier in my process, but I assured her that the Nutritional Yeast was surely enough at 630% B12 in it. NOT! Big ups to Asabi for being there throughout my ENTIRE process of healing, giving me guidance and insight when it comes to food and medicine.

There was a period during my healing process when I did not feel strong enough to walk on my own. To the eye, I could walk fine. Inside, my body felt weak, though. I could not tell what was wrong. One day, I got a spiritual download that told me to address the parasites in my body with a product called "Para 3" that I got from my nutritionist. Lo and behold, two days after getting those Para 3 drops into my system, after the incident, I could feel my body's strength! That uneasiness inside my body must have been caused by a block party the parasites were having inside of me. Before taking the drops, it felt like my equilibrium was off. The presence of parasites was also indicated by patches of dry skin on my elbows and right foot. I had tightness in my fingers, too. Come to find out, the skin eruptions and joint stiffness were all symptoms of having parasites in my system. I'm not into killing, yet being a host for those little varmints was going to end immediately!

Another body talking point was tremoring INSIDE my body. I only felt that sensation when I laid down. I discovered that it usually meant I needed to eliminate waste from my body. Once I'd eliminate, the sensation would go away, and I was able to go back to sleep. I looked up tremors inside the body and found that a B12 deficiency could be the culprit. I got B12 drops right away. After about a week or so, the tremors went away and I was able to have good sound sleep.

At another point during my healing process, I was experiencing twitching all over my body. I felt twitching in my face, in my legs, in my chest, just all over the place. Come to find out that I was deficient in Magnesium. One of the tests done by the doctors revealed that I was deficient in Magnesium, yet I was never told to remedy it. I listened to a higher power, and without a moment's pause after my research, I got Magnesium from the health food store, and those twitches ceased as well.

At one point in my healing process, my daughter pointed out that my teeth looked grey. I went in for closer inspection, and my teeth were looking BLACK on the backside. My teeth got heavily stained from the BLUEBERRIES I blended in my morning and evening smoothies.

I ended up getting a special charcoal-infused toothpaste called "Talk," at Trnscnd Wellness ([https://ourwellness888.com](https://ourwellness888.com)). I love the way the toothpaste makes my teeth feel, and they began to get back to the desired white teeth I had before the blueberries.

My body also experienced a variety of high blood pressure phenomena. I could always tell when my pressure was rising because I experienced a tight feeling in my eyes. They'd also start to water. The body talk that let me know my pressure was rising for sure was a slight burning sensation at the bottom of my right foot. That feeling was always accompanied by a similar sensation in my right calf. Those feelings let me know that I had to either eat something to address the issue or, in the worst case, take blood pressure medicine. We'll read more about the remedies in the food section coming up.

## YOU'RE THE HOST OF THE SHOW

There are about 6 different definitions for the word "host", yet I will share just two that are relevant here.

**Host - noun**

1. a master of ceremonies, moderator, or interviewer for a television or radio program, podcast, online chat space, or the like.

2. Biology - a living organism that is the source of nutrition for a parasite

We are going to jump all in the specialized Biology definition. Let's talk about OUR BODIES as a source of nutrition for parasites! Now just hold your horses. Many folks don't even want to entertain the idea of little organisms living in their bodies. Well, there are signs galore that point to just that:

**General Symptoms:**
1. **Abdominal pain**
2. **Cramping**
3. **Diarrhea**
4. **Constipation**
5. **Bloating**
6. **Excessive gas**
7. **Nausea**
8. **Vomiting**
9. **Fatigue or weakness**
10. **Unexplained weight loss**
11. **Itchy skin**
12. **Itchy anus (particularly with pinworms)**
13. **Rashes**
14. **Skin lesions**
15. **Fever**
16. **Chills**
17. **Sweating**

18. **Muscle or joint pain**

19. **Headache**

20. **Dizziness**

21. **Dehydration (due to diarrhea)**

22. **Dark circles under eyes**

23. **Loss of appetite**

24. **Swelling in the abdomen (due to bloating or worms)**

25. **Change in stool color (e.g., pale or bloody stool)**

**Specific Symptoms Related to Different Parasites:**

1.  **Visible worms in stool** (e.g., tapeworms or roundworms)

2.  **Presence of tapeworm segments in stool**

3.  **Coughing (often due to lung migration of worms)**

4.  **Liver enlargement (due to liver flukes or amoebas)**

5.  **Painful urination or blood in urine** (in case of urinary parasites like schistosomiasis)

6.  **Increased appetite** (common in some intestinal worms like tapeworms)

7.  **Confusion or disorientation** (can occur with certain brain-infecting parasites, like toxoplasmosis)

8.  **Severe abdominal bloating after eating** (due to giardia or other intestinal parasites)

9.  **Jaundice (yellowing of skin/eyes)** (may occur with liver-infecting parasites)

10. **Pale or anemic appearance** (due to blood loss from hookworms or other parasitic worms)

11. **Difficulty breathing** (caused by parasitic larvae migrating through the lungs)

12. **Night sweats** (commonly associated with malaria)

13. **Sleep disturbances or insomnia** (due to discomfort or itching from pinworms)

14. **Persistent cough** (sometimes caused by lung-dwelling parasites like strongyloides)

15. **Bloody stools** (due to severe intestinal infection or damage caused by parasites like Entamoeba histolytica)

16. **Grinding teeth (Bruxism)** Bruxism is typically caused by stress or anxiety, but it can also be linked to parasitic infections, especially if the parasites cause discomfort or disrupt sleep.

17. **Drooling** Toxoplasmosis: This parasitic infection (caused by the *Toxoplasma gondii* parasite) sometimes affects the brain, causing neurological symptoms such as confusion, lack of coordination, and even drooling.

18. **Joint Pain**
    **Migration through tissues**: Some parasites, like **strongyloides** and **trichinosis**, can migrate through body tissues, causing irritation, muscle, and joint pain as they pass through the body.

**Chronic inflammation**: Infections like **schistosomiasis** and **filariasis** can cause chronic inflammatory responses that affect the joints and lead to swelling, pain, and stiffness.

Okay, all of that above is research in and of itself. What I have to share is how much better I felt once I addressed the issue of having parasites in MY body. My personal first encounter dealt with having my knee go out while sprinting to catch a bus just ahead of me. I did not fall to the ground, yet when I got off the bus, I could not walk. I went to the hospital that same day and got X-rays done. The doctors said they did not see anything in the X-rays and that I should just R.I.C.E., which means Raise, use Ice, Compress, and Elevate my leg. You know why they didn't see anything? BECAUSE BONES ARE SEEN IN X-RAYS, NOT PARASITES. It wasn't until I told my Nutritionist about these joint experiences and other effects I was having in my life at the time, that she schooled me about what was really happening. At one point, I would feel a sensation that would travel from my head and down into my right leg. When that happened…it happened about 3 or 4 times…my leg from the knee to the ankle would give out and I could no longer stand on that leg. I would have to fall on the nearest couch or chair to avoid falling to the floor. After about 30 seconds, I would be able to stand again. The other physical manifestations I experienced at that time were elbows with scaly skin, and grating my teeth while sleeping.

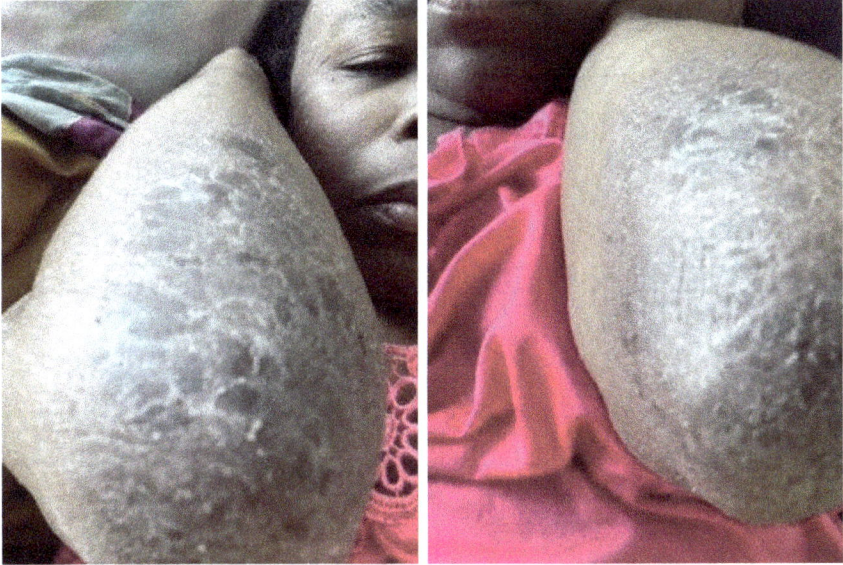

I would grate my teeth so hard that I would wake myself up at night doing so. Because of my scaly skin and joint discomfort, I inquired about what sounded like it could be Psoriatic Arthritis. That's when my Nutritionist gently said with firm confidence, "Oh no, you have parasites."

I began taking a product called "Para 3" and saw almost immediate results. I have not been grating my teeth anymore, there's no more pain in the joints of my fingers, my knees do not give out anymore, and I definitely do not feel sensations of anything moving through my body at all. I am on the last vestiges of clearing up the skin on my elbows and started to take a product called "Para 2" to do so. There are so many types of parasites, and the key is to find out what they are and address them accordingly. I saw a video that mentioned how pumpkin seeds PARALYZE parasites, and I suuurely make sure I sprinkle them over every salad I eat. Ask your doctor or nutritionist about testing for parasites. You will feel an inner strength when you handle them and have better control of your overall bodily functions.

## WHAT HEALTH FEELS LIKE

I am extremely thankful for getting a sense of what REAL good health feels like. I said earlier that I hardly knew people who lived good, healthy lives, so where was my frame of reference? How I know I am healthier feels closest to what I deem freedom feels like. When the body is going through challenges, some parts of the body don't work at their best. The opposite word that matches that ultimate feeling I'm talking about is INVINCIBLE. The definition for that word says, "Incapable of being conquered, defeated or subdued." Have you ever felt that way? Would you like to feel that way? I LOVE feeling that way! The energy is right, and there are no obstacles in sight when I feel invincible. Imagine a life that's worry-free. With the absence of body worries, I can focus on enjoying things. My attention goes right to creating things. It's challenging to create when hardship is taking all the attention. Imagine breathing easily, exercising without pain, thinking without brain fog, or lacking memory. Write the abilities you'd like to strengthen through having better health.

---

---

---

# WHAT I DON'T WANT

There are a ton of things we can do to make ourselves feel our best. THINKING about doing them is as far as we get sometimes. Here is a list below explaining what I DON'T want to experience:

- Tingling in my toes
- Headaches
- Pain in my chest
- Dizziness
- Pain in my knees
- Feeling weak
- Fear of walking unaccompanied
- Shortness of breath
- Constipation
- Bad eyesight
- Taking medicine that harms me while it "helps" me
- Injecting insulin daily
- Fatigue
- Nausea
- A body full of parasites
- Cravings created by organisms living inside my body
- Skin eruptions
- Arthritic-type pain in my joints
- Black teeth

- Odor from an unclean internal body

- High blood pressure

- Repeated trips to the hospital

- Too much urination

- Low energy

- Weight gain

- Unhappiness

- Lack of Purpose

- Tiredness

What are some of the things you DON'T want to experience?
Write them below:

_____

_____

_____

_____

_____

_____

_____

_____

_____

_____

# BLOOD PRESSURE & STRESS

I've never had to be this aware of stress in my life…ever! Both my strokes were stress-induced, along with high sugar. Now in life, it seems that the smallest upsets affect me greatly, and my blood pressure rises immediately to alarming levels. This makes it so that I must minimize bad news and people in my life who don't make me feel good. I've also had to learn methods of calming myself down. The 4-7-8 breathing helps. And, I have become extremely aware of foods that manage and lower blood pressure.

Learning about my adrenal glands was important for me to know. These are the glands that are directly related to stress.

Check out this information:

The adrenal glands are small, but mighty — they sit on top of your kidneys (like little hats) and play a huge role in managing your body's response to stress, energy levels, and hormone balance. Each gland has two main parts, and they each handle different jobs:

## Adrenal Gland Functions

### 1. Adrenal Cortex (outer layer)

Produces vital hormones for everyday body function:

- **Cortisol** – the "stress hormone":
  - Regulates metabolism
  - Helps control blood sugar

- o Reduces inflammation

- o Helps your body respond to stress

- **Aldosterone -**

  - o Regulates blood pressure by balancing sodium and potassium.

- **Androgens (sex hormones):**

  - o Contribute to the development of secondary sex characteristics, especially in women (like pubic hair and libido)

## 2. Adrenal Medulla (inner core)

Kicks in during fight or flight situations:

- Produces adrenaline **(epinephrine) and noradrenaline (norepinephrine)**

  - o Increases heart rate.

  - o Raises blood pressure.

  - o Boosts energy and alertness.

  - o Expands air passages in the lungs.

The adrenal glands help regulate:

- Stress response

- Energy production

- Blood pressure

- Metabolism

- Sex hormone balance

Here's how we can support our Adrenal Glands naturally:

## 1. Prioritize Quality Sleep

- Aim for 7–9 hours of restful sleep.

- Stick to a regular sleep schedule.

- Avoid screens and stimulants before bed.

## 2. Eat a Balanced, Nutrient-Rich Diet

- Focus on whole foods: veggies, fruits, lean proteins, healthy fats.

- Include complex carbs like sweet potatoes or brown rice (especially helpful for cortisol regulation).

- Limit caffeine and sugar — they can spike cortisol and exhaust your adrenals over time.

- Include adrenal-supportive nutrients:

    o   Vitamin C (peppers, citrus, berries)

    o   B Vitamins (leafy greens, eggs, legumes)

    o   Magnesium (avocados, nuts, dark chocolate)

    o   Zinc (pumpkin seeds, lentils, shellfish)

## 3. Manage Stress Effectively

- Try deep breathing, meditation, journaling, or yoga.

- Get out into nature or do something creative!

- Take breaks throughout the day — don't run on empty!

## 4. Stay Hydrated

- Dehydration can stress your adrenal glands.

- Add a pinch of sea salt or try coconut water for natural electrolytes (especially if you're feeling lightheaded or burnt out).

## 5. Exercise – But Don't Overdo It

- Gentle movement like walking, stretching, swimming, or yoga is great.

- Avoid overtraining, especially if you're already feeling exhausted — intense workouts can spike cortisol too much.

## 6. Adaptogenic Herbs (with caution & guidance)

Some herbs may help support adrenal health and stress resilience:

- Ashwagandha – calming and cortisol-balancing

- Rhodiola – energy-boosting and stress-fighting

- Holy basil (Tulsi) – soothing for the nervous system

*Talk to a healthcare provider or herbalist before starting herbs, especially if you have high blood pressure, are pregnant, or are on medications.*

## 7. Laugh, Connect, and Have Fun

- Social connection and joy are underrated adrenal boosters.

- Even 15 minutes of something you enjoy daily can make a huge difference.

# 4-7-8 BREATHING

When it came to addressing my blood pressure levels, I researched and even found a new method to breathe to calm my body. I learned that you must breathe through your nose for 4 counts. Then you hold your breath for 7 counts. The third step is to breathe out through your mouth, emptying your abdomen for 8 counts. For me, this breathing process worked immediately when I felt my heart beating fast or pounding. By the second or third time doing this cycle, I could feel my heart rate slowing down. This created a heightened calm in me, and I could relax better. When you do your own research, it is recommended that you do this five times to be effective. I personally would do these cycles as many times as my body allowed. I even caught myself falling asleep mid-breath and got awakened by a gasp for air. Lol. I am working to make it a habit to do these breaths during the day and not just in times of challenge. Our internal organs need oxygen to function properly, and deep breathing is a great way to be in total control of making sure the organs get it. The research I found below is spot on and describes my experience exactly:

### 4-7-8- breathing:

- **Improves sleep**

A lot of people use it to fall asleep faster. Slowing your breath and holding it like this can reduce anxiety and slow your heart rate, helping your body wind down.

- **Reduces anxiety and stress**

That deep, controlled breathing sends a signal to your brain that you're safe and everything's okay. It helps take the edge off when you're feeling anxious or overwhelmed.

- **Lowers blood pressure and heart rate**

With consistent practice, it can help reduce blood pressure and promote cardiovascular health by improving oxygen flow and lowering stress hormones.

- **Improves focus**

The controlled nature of breath helps clear your mind, making it easier to concentrate or reset during a busy or hectic day.

Make this a breathing habit, no matter what your condition is. Your body will thank you!

## WASHING THE INSIDE

What would happen if you didn't bathe or shower for decades? What would you expect? Would you smell? Might new critters appear on your body? If you didn't wash your body, you would surely tell the difference between how you feel when you're clean. Being that dirty would cause alarm. So let me ask a question. You only have one body, right? Second question - How often do you clean the INSIDE of your body? If the answer is very little or never, then imagine what the condition is INSIDE your body. Goodness gracious! I'm over 50 years wise and I have made efforts to clean the inside of my body maybe twice. And that was only through colonics, meaning only my intestines were directly affected.

Now that I have a higher consciousness of the ENTIRETY of my body, I am aware of the need to clean out my arteries and parts of the body that have a buildup of plaque and other substances in my arteries, teeth, colon, and even in my brain. Getting labs done in a hospital or working with a nutritionist like I do can give you clues to areas of the body you should give greater attention to. Feeling healthy is waaaay more pleasant than pushing through pain and discomfort. Both pain and discomfort in the body are usually a sign of something malfunctioning. Mucus, inflammation, and rashes are also signs of needing to clean out the inside of your body. Get a clue to what YOU need to do to improve the inner climate of your body.

Now, I can feel a stronger heartbeat, clearer skin, regular bowel movements, and greater alertness because of tending to my body's inner state. It's easy to ignore because we can't SEE unwanted substances like we do when we get a smudge on our skin. It's much more detrimental not to clean our insides, letting unwanted conditions grow, fester, and accumulate over time. Don't wait till it's too late to handle!

## DEFICIENCY

One area of health you never really hear people talk about is focusing on what we're deficient in. That means what we lack in our system, but sorely need for normal bodily functioning. What's usually done is that we get sick, and we're prescribed something to address the illness. What's missing first is the idea, "What **SHOULD** the body look and FEEL like in its natural state?" Once you're clear about the body's optimal state, then you can address what you should be looking for in foods, vitamins, and minerals.

As Westerners, we seem to be deficient in Vitamins K2, D3, and B12, as well as minerals like Magnesium. My concern for my own personal deficiencies came from feeling weak, not feeling strong enough to walk alone, tremoring in my feet, and body twitching in various parts of my body. I would then go look up what the symptoms of those things meant, and the foods associated with treating those symptoms. When I took a parasite cleanse, Magnesium and B12, I started to feel strong again. Taking Magnesium Glycinate helped that foot tremor to subside and go away. When I added B12 to my daily regimen, I absolutely felt stronger, and the twitching in my face seemed to subside and go away in a matter of days.

My bad cholesterol level was too high, and I chose to add Sunflower Lecithin to my morning and evening smoothies to remedy my cholesterol issue. The doctor told me that I started with my bad cholesterol (LDL) at 203mg/dL, then it went down to 124mg/dL, and my third reading was down to 103mg/dL. The desired number is 70mg/dL. With my daily intake of sunflower lecithin and "Cholesterol Secret: Blood Lipid Formula," I should be in that range when I get to my next doctor visit.

## B Vitamin Deficiency

B Vitamins do a lot and are essential for healthy neurology. With such a heavy emphasis on needing a "mental health day" these days, knowing what I am about to say is crucial! There was a time about 3 or 4 years ago when I was experiencing some version of anxiety. I started to feel claustrophobic in elevators. I felt weird and closed in when going into the train tunnels in the subways. I even had to have my daughter take me for walks to try and acknowledge things near and far and get some space. Then one day, I got a download from the Creator that said, "Look up B Vitamin deficiency." When I looked it up, boy, I saw so much of what I was experiencing.

My friend Asabi told me to purchase Nutritional Yeast to eat, as it is full of B vitamins, and she knew I wasn't a pill taker. Sure enough, it worked! I would take about a teaspoon of Nutritional Yeast and put it under my tongue. Right away, I would feel a calming sensation in my head, and after a few minutes, I'd simply drink it all down and let the rest of my digestive system have at it. From that point on, I always took nutritional yeast when I felt any odd head manifestations.

Not too long thereafter, my favorite DJ, Duane Powell, sent me an article showing that doctors in Asia discovered that B vitamin deficiency was related to anxiety and depression. Look it up! It's true.

**This is some of what I found:**

"…there is evidence linking B vitamin deficiency to anxiety and depression, particularly B12, B6, and B9 (folate). B vitamins are crucial for brain function and neurotransmitter synthesis, and deficiencies can impair mood and mental health. Vitamin B12, for example, is involved in the production of neurotransmitters that regulate mood, and low levels have been associated with depression and poor cognitive function."

Deficiencies in B12 can lead to psychological problems, ranging from mild depression or anxiety to more severe conditions like confusion and dementia.

## RESTORING MY BLOOD

Eating dark green leafy food is a sure-fire way of replenishing blood. *How?* Eating dark green leafy vegetables can help add to and support the health of your blood, particularly by contributing to the production of red blood cells and supporting overall circulatory health. But you can tell by one simple fact.

Chlorophyll is like the blood of plants. It closely resembles our red blood cells. Hemoglobin is the pigment that gives our blood its red color, as well as its oxygen-carrying capacity. The hemoglobin of the red blood cell and the Chlorophyll of the plant are virtually identical in molecular structure.

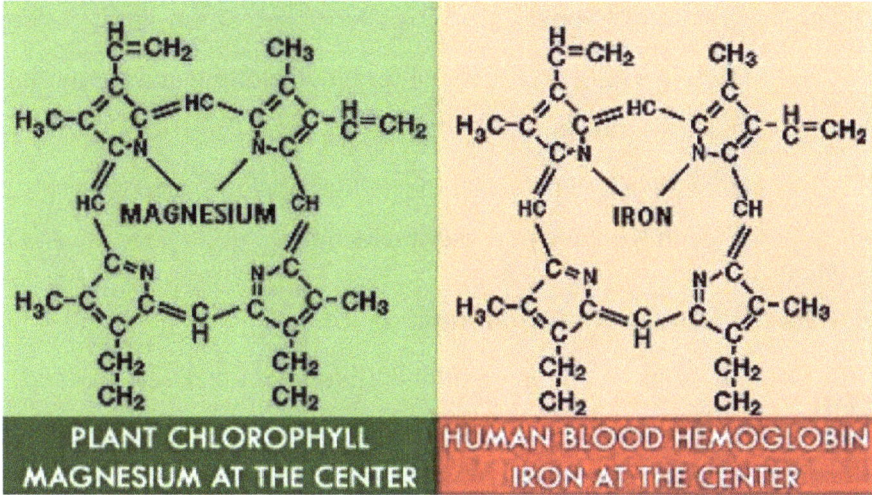

PLANT CHLOROPHYLL — MAGNESIUM AT THE CENTER / HUMAN BLOOD HEMOGLOBIN — IRON AT THE CENTER

I loved it when I found out this fact! This makes the need to add green leafy vegetables to our diet so evident. They are a part of my daily food intake. If for nothing else, we can experience replenished, healthy blood in our system by eating this way. You've got to love science!

Green leafy vegetables—like spinach, kale, collard greens, and Swiss chard—have a significant positive impact on blood health due to their rich nutritional profile. Here are some other facts supporting the use of green food to improve our human blood:

### 1. Increase in Red Blood Cell Production

- **Rich in folate (vitamin B9)**: Essential for red blood cell formation.

- **Iron content** (especially in spinach): Helps make hemoglobin, the protein in red blood cells that carries oxygen.

## 2. Improved Blood Clotting

- **High in vitamin K**: Crucial for blood clotting and preventing excessive bleeding.

- *Note*: People on blood thinners like warfarin need to monitor vitamin K intake to avoid interactions.

## 3. Detoxification & Anti-inflammatory Effects

- Chlorophyll and antioxidants (like lutein and beta-carotene) help detox the blood and reduce oxidative stress, lowering inflammation.

## 4. Blood Pressure and Circulation Support

- Nitrates (especially in leafy greens like arugula and spinach) help dilate blood vessels, improving blood flow and reducing blood pressure.

## 5. Balanced Blood Sugar Levels

- Fiber content helps stabilize blood sugar, reducing spikes and crashes—important for managing or preventing diabetes.

# ELIMINATING WASTE

There is a lot of waste that needs to leave the body. If you have a protruding belly, that is partially a sign of backed-up waste in your intestines. While stretching can be used for maintaining a lot of great bodily functions, I learned that stretching helps to eliminate waste from the body almost instantly. A man who worked at the university I attended told me to stretch as high as I could towards the sky in the morning when I woke up. He said that the stretching would elongate the intestines and make elimination easier. He was right. Then I learned that if you have a small foot stool in your bathroom, and your knees are raised close to your chest, you can experience immediate relief and elimination.

Lastly, and what I feel works the best, is the reaching over the shoulder stretch while you're sitting on the toilet. I just stumbled on this stretch and have been using it ever since. I take my left arm and stretch it to reach over my right shoulder. I then take my right hand and press the arm further over my shoulder. This move makes me eliminate immediately. And if I twist my waist to the right in the process…oooo doggy does this help the process. No constipation in sight!

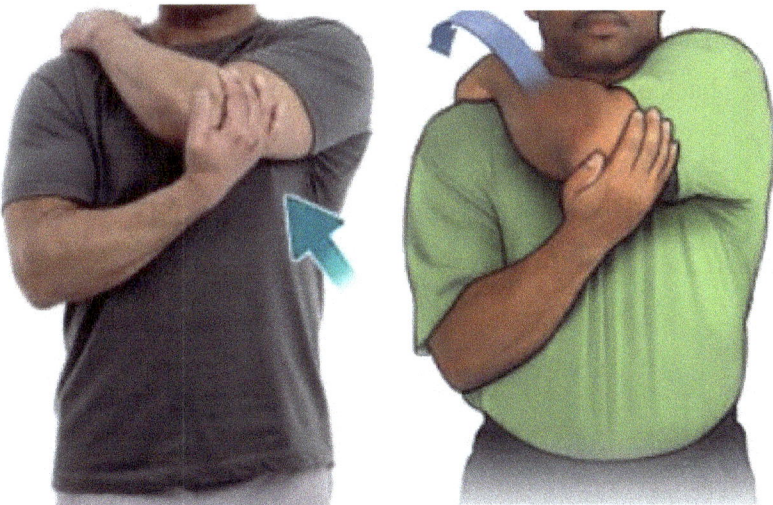

*Push the arm over the shoulder further for immediate elimination relief.*

My ability to eliminate waste from my body became important because of how my head would feel, believe it or not. I noticed that when I felt uneasiness or fogginess in my brain, it usually meant that it was time to go to the restroom. Sure enough, once I eliminated them, I'd feel a clearing of those sensations in my brain. During my healing process, I have become more aware of the tie between what's going on in my brain and how it's connected to what's in my gut or intestines. The brain and intestines even look similar. I chose to look and see if there was, in fact, a connection between the gut and brain, and this is what I found:

## GUT-BRAIN CONNECTION: HOW IT WORKS

### 1. The Vagus Nerve: The Superhighway

- The vagus nerve is the main nerve pathway that sends signals back and forth between your brain and gut.

- It affects things like:
    - Digestion
    - Heart rate
    - Mood
    - Stress response

### 2. Neurotransmitters Made in the Gut

- Your gut produces many of the same chemicals your brain uses to regulate mood:
    - **Serotonin**: ~90% is made in your gut!

- o **Dopamine**
- o **GABA**
- Imbalances in the gut can influence anxiety, depression, and cognitive function.

## 3. Microbiome: The Tiny Brain Helpers

- Your gut hosts trillions of bacteria (gut microbiota) that play a role in:
  - o Neurotransmitter production
  - o Immune regulation
  - o Inflammation
  - o Nutrient absorption
- A healthy microbiome = better brain health.

## 4. Inflammation & the Immune System

- **Chronic gut inflammation** (from poor diet, stress, dysbiosis) can release **pro**-inflammatory cytokines that affect the brain and lead to issues like:
  - o Brain fog
  - o Mood swings
- Neurodegeneration
  The gut is home to **70–80% of your immune system**, so gut health directly impacts brain resilience.

## 5. Stress Affects Digestion

- Ever had "butterflies in your stomach" or felt sick when nervous?

- Stress and anxiety can slow digestion, increase acid, and worsen conditions like IBS or leaky gut.

- The brain can trigger gut symptoms—and vice versa.

## When Gut Health Influences the Brain

- Dysbiosis (imbalance in gut bacteria) is linked to:
  - Depression
  - Anxiety
  - ADHD
  - Alzheimer's & Parkinson's (emerging research)

## When Brain Health Influences the Gut

- Stress and trauma can cause:
  - IBS (irritable bowel syndrome)
  - SIBO (small intestinal bacterial overgrowth)
  - Appetite changes
  - Nutrient absorption issues

## What Supports a Healthy Gut-Brain Axis?

- **Probiotics & Prebiotics** (fermented foods, fiber-rich veggies)
- **Omega-3s** (flax, chia, fish oil)
- **Stress management** (breathwork, meditation, exercise)
- **Hydration & Sleep**
- **Avoiding ultra-processed foods and excess sugar**
  Your gut and brain are in constant conversation. When your gut is happy and balanced, your brain tends to follow. And when your mind is calm and nourished, digestion and microbiome health benefit too.

## READ LABELS

I've always taught my daughter to read the labels of foods while growing up. This way, she was young and aware of the foods she chose to eat. She even stopped adults from giving her food that wasn't in line with how she was raised. Now let's talk about my own reading of labels…present time! I am a label-reading hawk since my last and final stroke incident. As of recent, I loved a condiment and did not pay specific attention to what it was made up of. I was dousing my salad with this condiment with a fervor because I loved it so much. What I didn't read on that label was the SIZE I should have been using with all that dousing. It had 140 grams of sodium PER TEASPOON. The way I was using that stuff, I probably had about six or seven teaspoons applied to my food! No wonder my blood pressure was going into the 200s at night! Once I figured out the problem, not only did I obviously stop using that condiment, but my blood pressure started trending down, too.

If the labels of your food contain a list of items you can't even pronounce, first and foremost, look those things up. Second, consider whether you should be eating things you can't pronounce or even know what they are.

## FOOD AS MEDICINE

The five major goals I have in life right now are to keep my blood sugar and blood pressure levels controlled and in the proper range for good health, improve my neurological health and my cholesterol, and maintain a healthy gut environment. When you keep reading, you'll overstand WHY I eat what I currently eat. I am a firm believer that everything we need to live well was provided by the Most High. I can wholeheartedly say that food has become my true medicine during my time of healing. Many supplements claim that you can take them and eat the foods you've always wanted to eat. Well, I have news for you…that hasn't even been you wanting those foods. And there's no way that highly processed foods that were not naturally made by God are designed to enhance the body. Don't fool yourself. Those sugary foods that people tell you, "you're allowed to have a treat…" are really a trick.

Before having my seizure and second stroke, I knowingly ate other things I knew were not some help to my body…even being a "vegan." I was diagnosed in late 2008 with Diabetes. I learned that breads, pastas, and wheat products were not a friend to me. When I had my first stroke, my diet consisted of a TON of Chinese food, fast food restaurant fries, Garlic Nan bread from the Indian restaurant, and tall icy glasses of apple juice. I didn't know about those starches turning to sugar. I wasn't aware of the sugar content of processed apple juice or my orange juice/cranberry cocktail mixes. I just thought it was enough not to drink sodas. Eating starches is surely a thing when you don't eat meat. They add heaviness to the meal, and you don't feel as hungry. Little did I know the WHY of my hunger. I'd learn later that there were organisms inside of me that were craving the food I loved and not really cravings coming from ME.

I eat differently since my incident in August 2024. Yes, I have been a vegan since 1990, yet not eating cooked food was way off the radar. I enjoyed cooked food and dining too much to even consider not eating any food that wasn't cooked. Not eating meat for so long, I came across cuisine made specifically from raw preparation. I liked some of the cheeses made from nuts and such. More than anything, I enjoyed the way I felt when I ate raw food. I just never made time to prepare raw cuisine myself. I wasn't willing to spend the time to soak beans and blend nuts and other processes used to create that good food. Well, now in a new unit of time, I do a whole lot of the above and more.

My newly developed lifestyle entails very little cooked food. I only cook my quinoa and my tofu. These days, when my body has to digest cooked foods, it overworks, and my blood sugar seems to rise. My heart beats stronger, and I can even feel my pulse in my fingertips. So now I enjoy a nutrient-rich diet, mostly raw, with foods that I KNOW are enhancing me. You don't have to be like me and eat the foods I choose to eat. I will share them with you, though. You just may see something in your health you want to clear up or get rid of. I believe that the reason people don't aim for a healthier life is because they've never really seen one. I say forget that and FEEL it for yourself.

My daily meal has come down to one salad a day. Now this is no diet or anything. It's simply what my body calls for. It seldom wants much else.

I eat one salad a day that consists of the following:

There is usually a mixed spring salad, arugula, romaine lettuce, cilantro, spinach, fresh garlic, tri-color quinoa, red onions, pumpkin seeds, walnuts, apples, sunflower seeds, lentils, olive tapenade, cucumber, chickpeas, apple cider vinegar, avocados, tofu, toasted sesame oil, fresh squeezed lemon juice, and whatever spices I want to use. As a treat, I put "Lemon Avocado Sauce" by *Veggie Brunch LLC* on as a dressing. This is an olive oil-based sauce and is deeeeelishious! This salad lasts as my meal for the entire day. This is not a special diet, simply what my body began to accept as a norm. My personal process has been to look at the effect I want on my body and find the food, vitamins, and minerals that contribute toward creating that effect. Here is the breakdown of what I apply to my food life.

## Celery Juice - 16 oz every morning

I look forward to the effects celery juice has on me every morning. It serves as a natural medicine for me. Celery juice brings my blood pressure numbers down in the morning substantially! This is the very first food I ingest before ANYTHING, daily. The key is to drink it on an empty stomach for the best results. Here are some facts as to why that is.

Celery juice may help lower blood pressure due to its **phthalides**, potassium content, anti-inflammatory properties, and hydration benefits.

## Phthalides (Plant Compounds)

- Celery contains a compound called phthalides, which is thought to play a key role in reducing blood pressure. Phthalides can help relax the muscles in and around blood vessels, which promotes vasodilation (the widening of blood vessels). This relaxation of the blood vessels can lead to improved blood flow and lower blood pressure.

- Phthalides also stimulate the production of certain enzymes that help to reduce blood pressure and maintain healthy circulation.

One day, I experienced higher levels of my blood pressure late at night, so I made celery juice before I called the ambulance to come get me and take me to the hospital. My pressure was at 250! By the time I got in the ambulance, about 20 minutes later, the pressure went down to 190. When I got to the hospital, another 20 minutes later, my pressure went down to 166. This was all after drinking the celery juice. The medicine I took did not work effectively at that time, which is what made me make the juice. We love you, celery juice!

People have asked me if they can just EAT celery. I simply tell them that I don't know what it's like to EAT a whole bunch of celery. All I know is that the pack a day I JUICE in my juicer gives me 16oz of celery juice to drink. This amount has made my blood pressure go down from 150 to 130 in about an hour. I use this juice to set the tone for my day, and I work to maintain my pressure throughout the day NATURALLY.

## Eating Grapefruit

I learned in my research that eating grapefruit brings down blood pressure. It surely does! I have not noticed the same numerical decrease that I see when I drink celery juice, yet I feel the physical effects of high blood pressure levels subside when I eat them. Some of the high blood pressure physical effects have been a tightness behind my eyes and slight watering. This is usually accompanied by a slight tingling in my right calf and the bottom of my right foot, near the toes. Once I consumed just half a grapefruit, I felt those feelings go away.

It's advised not to eat grapefruit at the same time as you take blood pressure medicine. Apparently, the grapefruit will cancel out the effectiveness of the medicine. At the time of writing this book, I take my blood pressure medicine in the evening before I go to bed. Therefore, I will eat the grapefruit in the middle of the day. If I feel any high blood pressure discomforts in the middle of the night, I simply go eat a ½ a grapefruit and go back to bed, having knocked out those unwanted sensations. While taking too much medication scares me, I feel great knowing I can munch on grapefruit as much as I want, without any side effects or harm to my body.

## Water and Hydration

I learned that being hydrated is important when trying to maintain a healthy blood pressure range. Most people just think it's about drinking a lot of water. Well, as you'll read below, full hydration has to do with what's in the water, too. Hydration Helps Maintain Normal Blood Pressure

- Water makes up most of your blood volume.
  - When you're well-hydrated, your blood flows more easily and your heart doesn't have to work as hard to pump it.
  - This keeps blood pressure within a healthy range.
- Dehydration can reduce blood volume.
  - Less fluid in your bloodstream means the heart has to pump harder, which can temporarily raise blood pressure.
  - Or in some cases, dehydration can cause low blood pressure due to reduced volume, leading to dizziness or fainting.
- Blood pressure isn't just about how much water you drink— it's also about electrolyte balance.

**Sodium:**
- Too much sodium pulls water into the bloodstream, increasing blood volume and raising blood pressure.
- If you're dehydrated and consuming a lot of salt, it can worsen hypertension.

**Potassium:**
- Potassium helps relax blood vessels and balance sodium levels, which helps lower blood pressure.

- Staying hydrated with potassium-rich fluids (like coconut water or eating bananas, avocados, spinach, etc.) helps support a healthy balance.

## 4-oz Smoothies and Supplements

4-oz smoothies are the second food source I add to my daily food journey. I do not swallow pills easily, so I blend up my supplements into a smoothie. I do one in the morning, about two or three hours after my celery juice. I cut my bananas into one-inch sections, and I freeze them, along with my other morning fruits. In a small blending container, I add about an inch high amount of almond milk. I then add approximately five blueberries, one blackberry, one strawberry, and a section of banana. I add a tablespoon of ceylon cinnamon (sugar control). I add a tablespoon of nutritional yeast (sugar control and tons of B vitamins). I add a tablespoon of flaxseed meal and a tablespoon of sunflower lecithin. I put in about a teaspoon of chia seeds and then all of my supplements. My supplements at the time of writing this section are:

> **AnxioCalm** - is a natural, non-drowsy supplement formulated to alleviate occasional anxiety, stress, and nervous tension. Developed by Terry Naturally (EuroPharma), it is suitable for both adults and children aged 4 and up. The primary active component in AnxioCalm is **EP107™**, a proprietary extract of *Echinacea angustifolia* (narrow-leaved coneflower). While echinacea is commonly associated with immune support, this

specific extract is standardized for unique alkamides and echinacosides, which have been clinically studied for their calming effects on the nervous system.

**Biotoxin Binder** - Biotoxin binders assist in removing harmful substances from the body, supporting overall detoxification efforts. By eliminating toxins that may disrupt the gut microbiome, these binders promote a healthy digestive system and bolster immune function.

**Bucco No. 25** - is an herbal liquid supplement developed by *Nestmann Pharma* and distributed in the U.S. by *Marco Pharma*. It's formulated to support kidney and urinary tract health, particularly in cases of subacute and chronic kidney conditions.

## Key Benefits

- **Diuretic Action**: Promotes urine flow to aid in flushing the urinary tract.

- **Protects Urinary Lining**: Helps maintain the health of the urinary tract's epithelial lining.

- **Anti-inflammatory & Antispasmodic**: May alleviate inflammation and spasms in the urinary system.

- **Kidney Stone Prevention**: Assists in preventing the formation of kidney stones.

- **Adrenal Support**: Provides mild stimulation to the adrenal glands.

- **Improved Renal Circulation**: Enhances blood flow within the kidneys.

- Some users have reported improvements in conditions like chronic kidney disease (CKD), bladder spasms, and urinary discomfort after using Bucco No. 25.

## Herbal Ingredients

Bucco No. 25 contains a blend of traditional herbs known for their urinary and kidney support:

> Buchu leaf, Rupturewort, Horsetail, White Willow bark, Licorice root, Peppermint leaf, Java Tea leaf, Juniper berry, Restharrow root, Common Bean shell, Birch leaf, Uva-Ursi leaf.

**Cardio Plus** - designed to support the healthy functioning of the heart and other muscles, as well as promote healthy coronary blood flow.

**Cataplex B2** - is a dietary supplement made by *Standard Process*, a company known for producing whole food-based supplements. Cataplex B2 is designed to support the nervous system and cardiovascular health, with a particular focus on the function of B-complex vitamins, especially vitamin B2 (riboflavin) and its associated nutrients.

**Cholesterol Secret Blood and Lipid Formula** is a liquid herbal supplement crafted by *Secrets of the Tribe*, designed to support healthy cholesterol levels and overall cardiovascular health. This alcohol-free tincture combines traditional herbs known for their potential benefits in lipid metabolism and heart health. ***It's made up of:***

| | |
|---|---|
| **Artichoke** | May help reduce high cholesterol levels and promote good cholesterol production. |
| **Astragalus** | Believed to support cardiovascular health and longevity. |
| **Hawthorn** | Used to improve cardiovascular system health, normalize blood pressure, and prevent hardening of arteries. |
| **Fennel** | Historically used for digestive health and may support overall cardiovascular well-being. |

**Core Berberine** - Berberine has been shown to lower blood sugar levels by improving insulin sensitivity and reducing glucose production in the liver.

**EZ Mag - E-Z Mg** is a plant-based, organic magnesium supplement developed to support individuals with inadequate dietary magnesium intake. It combines magnesium-rich ingredients like Swiss chard (beet leaf) and buckwheat. Essential for maintaining a healthy nervous system. Helps address magnesium deficiencies common in many diets. Provides an excellent source of vitamin K1 and iron, and a good source of magnesium.

**Hawthorn** - Hawthorn is often used to help with congestive heart failure (CHF) and mild heart rhythm disturbances. It can improve the heart's ability to pump blood more efficiently. It helps dilate blood vessels, improving blood flow and reducing strain on the heart.

**Hypothalmapath** – is a homeopathic combination formula for symptoms related to the endocrine and nervous systems. Communication between these two vital systems is accomplished by the hypothalamus via the pituitary gland. It's a natural supplement that supports the hypothalamus' function. It's often used in functional medicine to help balance hormones, support metabolism, and address chronic fatigue or adrenal issues. The hypothalamus and adrenal glands are interconnected through a key pathway called the hypothalamic-pituitary-adrenal (HPA) axis. The HPA axis plays a crucial role in the body's response to stress, regulating the release of hormones like cortisol and aldosterone from the adrenal glands.

Here are some of its purposes:

1. **Hormonal balance**
   Supports the hypothalamus, which helps regulate thyroid, adrenal, and reproductive hormones.

2. **Improved stress response**
   Supporting the HPA (hypothalamic-pituitary-adrenal) axis, may help with stress resilience and reduce cortisol imbalances.

3. **Better sleep and energy**
   May support circadian rhythm regulation, leading to improved sleep patterns and reduced fatigue.

4. **Appetite and metabolism support**
   Helps regulate signals for hunger and satiety, potentially aiding in healthy weight management.

5. **Mood stabilization**
   Can support neurotransmitter balance, possibly reducing anxiety or mood swings related to hormonal fluctuations.

6. **Support during detox or chronic illness protocols**
   Some practitioners use it as part of treatment for Lyme, mold illness, or chronic fatigue syndromes to rebalance neuroendocrine function.

**Lymphtone III** - Lymph-Tone III is designed to enhance the lymphatic system's ability to eliminate waste and toxins from the body.

**Magnesium -** Being deficient in Magnesium had a big effect on my not feeling strong. Once I started taking a magnesium supplement, my condition improved, and I felt better able to walk unaccompanied. Magnesium is an essential mineral that plays a key role in many important functions in the body. Here are some of its top benefits:

1. **Supports Muscle and Nerve Function**: Magnesium helps regulate muscle and nerve function. It is involved in transmitting nerve impulses and maintaining normal muscle function, which is important for preventing muscle cramps and spasms.

2. **Promotes Bone Health**: Magnesium works with calcium and vitamin D to support strong bones. It helps in the absorption of calcium and contributes to bone formation and strength.

3. **Regulates Blood Sugar Levels**: Magnesium helps regulate blood sugar levels and improve insulin sensitivity, which can be beneficial for those with type 2 diabetes or at risk for it.

4. **Heart Health**: Magnesium helps maintain normal heart rhythm and may help reduce the risk of heart disease by supporting blood pressure regulation. It also helps in reducing inflammation, which is a risk factor for heart disease.

5. **Improves Sleep**: Magnesium can help improve sleep quality by promoting relaxation and supporting the production of melatonin, the hormone responsible for regulating sleep.

6. **Reduces Anxiety and Stress**: Magnesium has been shown to have a calming effect on the nervous system, which can help reduce feelings of anxiety and stress.

7. **Supports Digestive Health**: Magnesium helps maintain normal bowel function by relaxing the muscles in the intestines, which can aid in preventing constipation.

8. **Relieves Headaches and Migraines**: Some studies suggest that magnesium deficiency may contribute to headaches and migraines, so getting adequate magnesium may help reduce the frequency and severity of these conditions.

9. **Supports Protein Synthesis and Energy Production**: Magnesium is involved in the production of ATP (adenosine triphosphate), which is the main energy carrier in cells. It also

plays a role in the synthesis of proteins and the production of DNA and RNA.

10. **Anti-Inflammatory Effects**: Magnesium has been shown to help reduce markers of inflammation in the body, which may be beneficial for those dealing with chronic inflammatory conditions.

Because magnesium is involved in so many vital processes, it's important to ensure you're getting enough through your diet or supplements if necessary. Foods rich in magnesium include leafy green vegetables, nuts, seeds, whole grains, and legumes.

**Neurotrophin PMG** - The PMG extracts in Neurotrophin PMG® are intended to promote the natural repair processes of brain cells, enhancing overall nervous system function.

**Potassium** - Potassium helps regulate the balance of fluids inside and outside of cells, ensuring they function properly. It's vital for maintaining a healthy cellular environment. Potassium helps counteract the effects of sodium, which can raise blood pressure. By balancing sodium levels, potassium helps lower high blood pressure, reducing the risk of heart disease and stroke. Potassium is essential for normal heart rhythm. It helps maintain electrical conductivity in the heart, reducing the risk of arrhythmias (irregular heartbeats). Potassium is a key electrolyte that helps regulate fluid balance in the body, preventing dehydration and helping maintain proper hydration levels. Potassium aids in the function of the kidneys by helping to balance the amount of water in the blood, which contributes to the proper excretion of waste through urine.

**Rauwolfia** - Rauwolfia is renowned for its ability to lower high blood pressure. The primary active compound, reserpine, helps reduce blood pressure by depleting norepinephrine and serotonin in the brain, leading to vasodilation and decreased heart rate. Rauwolfia has been used to alleviate symptoms of anxiety and stress. Its sedative properties can help calm the nervous system.

**Ribonucleic Acid (RNA)** - RNA is essential for making proteins. It's the messenger RNA (mRNA) that carries genetic info from DNA to the ribosomes, where proteins are built. No RNA = no proteins = no life. Some RNAs help detect and silence viruses in cells. For example, RNA interference (RNAi) can be used to shut down viral genes or faulty genes in diseases.

**Sea Moss Advanced**

*Sea Moss Advanced* by Infinite Age is a high-potency dietary supplement designed to support overall wellness, including energy levels, immune function, and digestive health. Each capsule combines three potent ingredients: Irish Sea Moss, Bladderwrack, and Burdock Root, offering a comprehensive blend of nutrients.

**Irish Sea Moss**: Rich in iodine, potassium chloride, and a variety of vitamins and minerals, it supports thyroid function, respiratory health, and immune system strength.

**Bladderwrack**: Contains fucoidan and fucoxanthin, compounds known for their anti-inflammatory and antioxidant properties, which may aid in weight management and digestive health.

**Burdock Root**: Acts as a prebiotic, promoting gut health and nutrient absorption, while also offering antioxidant benefits that support skin health and reduce inflammation.

**Spanish Black Radish** - Rich in glucosinolates, Spanish Black Radish aids in detoxification by stimulating bile production and promoting liver function. Packed with vitamin C, Spanish Black Radish strengthens the immune system and helps the body fight infections.

**Vitamin K** - Vitamin K2 helps regulate calcium in the body, ensuring it is deposited in bones and teeth rather than soft tissues like arteries. By supporting proper blood clotting and calcium regulation, vitamin K contributes to overall cardiovascular health.

**HERE ARE SOME GREAT FACTS ABOUT THE FOODS IN MY DAILY SMOOTHIE:**

**Almond Milk**

**1. Dairy-Free & Lactose-Free**

- Perfect for people with lactose intolerance, milk allergies, or those following a vegan diet.
- Gentle on digestion and doesn't cause bloating or gas like some dairy products can.

## 2. Low in Calories (Especially Unsweetened)

- Unsweetened almond milk has only 30–50 calories per cup, much lower than dairy milk or other plant milks.

- Great for weight management or low-calorie diets.

## 3. Heart-Healthy Fats

- Made from almonds, which contain monounsaturated fats— the same heart-healthy fats found in olive oil and avocados.

- These fats help lower bad LDL cholesterol and may support heart health.

## 4. Naturally Low in Sugar

- Unsweetened versions have little to no sugar—ideal for blood sugar balance, diabetics, or anyone reducing added sugar intake.

- Be cautious with sweetened or flavored varieties, which can contain added sugars.

## 5. Often Fortified with Bone-Boosting Nutrients

- Most commercial almond milks are fortified with:
  - Calcium (to match or exceed dairy levels)

- Vitamin D (essential for calcium absorption)

- Vitamin B12 (especially important for vegans)

- This makes almond milk a strong supporter of bone health and nerve function.

## 6. Hydrating and Easy on the Stomach

- Almond milk is mostly water, which helps you hydrate.

- It's also easier to digest than dairy for many people, with no casein or **whey** (common allergens in cow's milk).

## 7. Rich in Vitamin E (a powerful antioxidant)

Almonds are naturally high in vitamin E, which supports:

- Skin health
- Eye health
- Immune function
- Protection against oxidative stress

## 8. No Cholesterol or Saturated Fat

- A heart-smart option compared to whole dairy milk, which contains cholesterol and saturated fat.

- Also free from hormones or antibiotics that can sometimes be found in conventional dairy.

### Blueberries

Blueberries are tiny nutritional powerhouses packed with vitamins, antioxidants, and other health-boosting compounds. Whether you eat them fresh, frozen, dried, or in smoothies, they bring a lot to the table—literally and figuratively. Here are some of the benefits:

## 1. Rich in Antioxidants

- Blueberries are one of the highest antioxidant foods, particularly high in anthocyanins, which give them their deep blue-purple color.

- Antioxidants protect your cells from oxidative stress and free radical damage, which can lead to aging and chronic diseases.

## 2. Boost Brain Health

- Studies suggest that regular consumption of blueberries can improve memory, cognitive function, and may delay age-related mental decline.

- The antioxidants in blueberries help reduce inflammation in the brain and improve neuronal signaling.

## 3. Support Heart Health

- Blueberries may help lower **LDL cholesterol** and **blood pressure**, both of which are major risk factors for heart disease.

- They improve arterial flexibility and reduce oxidative damage to LDL particles, which protects the cardiovascular system.

## 4. Help Manage Blood Sugar

- Blueberries have a low glycemic index, meaning they don't spike your blood sugar like some other fruits.

- The fiber and polyphenols in blueberries help improve insulin sensitivity and support stable glucose levels, making them diabetic-friendly in moderation.

## 5. Fight Inflammation

- Chronic inflammation is at the root of many diseases (heart disease, diabetes, cancer), and blueberries are known to be natural anti-inflammatories.

## 6. Cancer-Fighting Potential

- Research shows that blueberries may slow the growth of cancer cells, especially in the breast, colon, and prostate.
- Their rich antioxidant profile helps protect DNA from damage and can support natural detoxification pathways.

## 7. Aid in Digestive Health

- Blueberries are a good source of fiber, which supports digestion and healthy gut bacteria.
- A healthy gut is essential for nutrient absorption, immune health, and mental clarity.

## 8. Protect Eye Health

- Blueberries contain lutein and zeaxanthin, compounds known to protect the retina from oxidative stress and reduce the risk of age-related macular degeneration (AMD).
- They may also help combat eye fatigue and support vision, especially in low-light conditions.

### 9. Boost Immune System

- Rich in vitamin C, vitamin K, and manganese, blueberries help boost the immune response and strengthen the body's defenses against illness.

### 10. Support Healthy Aging

- The polyphenols in blueberries help slow cellular aging and may help maintain skin elasticity, joint health, and brain vitality.

## Strawberries

Note: My daughter taught me to soak my strawberries in water until they're covered, then sprinkle baking soda over them. After that, I apply vinegar, and boy, does it start bubbling up. *What does this do?* It cleans those little puppies wonderfully! You'll surely be able to tell once you remove them from that washing bowl. Here are some of their benefits:

### 1. Rich in Antioxidants

- Loaded with vitamin C—even more than oranges per serving!
- Contain anthocyanins, ellagic acid, and quercetin, which help fight free radicals, slow aging, and protect against disease.

### 2. Support Heart Health

- May help lower blood pressure and improve cholesterol levels (especially LDL and triglycerides).

- Anti-inflammatory effects support healthy blood vessels and improve circulation.
- Studies link strawberry consumption to a reduced risk of heart disease.

## 3. Improve Blood Sugar Regulation

- Despite their sweetness, strawberries have a low glycemic index, meaning they don't spike blood sugar levels (why they are in my morning smoothie).
- High in fiber, which helps slow sugar absorption and supports insulin sensitivity.

## 4. Boost Brain Function

- Antioxidants in strawberries (especially anthocyanins) have been shown to improve memory and cognitive performance, particularly as we age.
- May help protect brain cells from oxidative stress and inflammation.

## 5. Anti-Cancer Properties

- Ellagic acid and other antioxidants may inhibit cancer cell growth and help detoxify potential carcinogens.
- Studies suggest strawberries may help reduce the risk of breast, colon, and esophageal cancers.

## 6. Reduce Inflammation

- Chronic inflammation is linked to many diseases—strawberries help lower inflammatory markers like CRP (C-reactive protein).

- Their anti-inflammatory effects may benefit people with arthritis or autoimmune conditions.

## 7. Support Digestion and Gut Health

- High in fiber, which aids digestion, promotes regularity, and supports a healthy microbiome.

- Fiber also supports appetite control and weight management.

## 8. Good for Skin and Teeth

- Vitamin C supports collagen production, helping maintain firm, youthful skin.

- Some people use crushed strawberries for natural teeth whitening, thanks to **malic acid** (though this should be done cautiously to avoid **enamel** damage).

## 9. Eye Health

- Rich in vitamin C, flavonoids, and phenolic compounds that help prevent cataracts, macular degeneration, and vision decline.

## Bananas

When I bring my bananas home, I cut them into one- or two-inch segments as I peel them. I then put them in a plastic bag before putting them in the freezer. Here are some of the bananas' benefits:

### 1. Natural Energy Booster

- Packed with natural sugars (glucose, fructose, and sucrose) + fiber, bananas provide a quick and sustained energy boost.
- Great as a pre- or post-workout snack.

### 2. Supports Heart Health

- High in potassium, a key mineral that helps:
  - **Lower blood pressure**
  - **Regulate heart rhythm**
  - **Balance sodium levels**
- Regular potassium intake is linked to a reduced risk of stroke and heart disease.

### 3. Aids Digestion

- Rich in dietary fiber, especially pectin, which helps:
  - Promote regular bowel movements
  - Relieve constipation
  - Feed good gut bacteria
- Resistant starch in greener bananas acts like a prebiotic, supporting gut health.

## 4. Helps Manage Blood Sugar

- Despite being sweet, bananas have a low to medium glycemic index, especially when they're slightly green.

- Fiber and resistant starch slow sugar absorption and improve insulin sensitivity, especially in unripe bananas.

## 5. Boosts Mood and Reduces Stress

- Contain tryptophan, which your body converts into serotonin, the "feel-good" neurotransmitter.

- Also high in vitamin B6, which supports mood regulation and brain health.

- Magnesium in bananas may help relax muscles and reduce anxiety.

## 6. Supports Muscle Function

- Potassium and magnesium help prevent muscle cramps, especially after exercise.

- Ideal for athletes or anyone with an active lifestyle.

## 7. Brain Health & Focus

- Vitamin B6 helps produce neurotransmitters like dopamine and serotonin.

- Glucose from bananas provides steady energy to the brain, improving focus and memory.

## 8. Rich in Antioxidants

- Contain dopamine and catechins, antioxidants that help:

- o Reduce oxidative stress

- o Support heart and brain health

- o Combat inflammation

## 9. Helps with Weight Management

- The fiber and resistant starch can promote fullness and help reduce overall calorie intake.

- A great naturally sweet, low-calorie snack (~105 calories per medium banana).

## Blackberries

Blackberries are delicious, juicy, and absolutely packed with nutrition. These dark-colored berries are loaded with antioxidants, fiber, vitamins, and plant compounds that support nearly every system in your body—from your brain to your heart to your gut.

## 1. Super High in Antioxidants

- Rich in anthocyanins (the dark purple pigment), which help fight oxidative stress and inflammation.

- Other antioxidants include vitamin C, vitamin E, and ellagic acid, which all help prevent cell damage and chronic disease.

## 2. Boosts Brain Health

- May slow cognitive decline and improve memory and motor skills.

- Antioxidants in blackberries reduce neuroinflammation and support communication between brain cells.

- Some studies suggest regular consumption can support aging brains and help protect against diseases like Alzheimer's.

## 3. Supports Heart Health

- High in fiber, potassium, and polyphenols that help:
  - Lower blood pressure
  - Reduce LDL (bad) cholesterol
  - Improve circulation
  - Strengthen blood vessels

## 4. Excellent for Digestive Health

- One cup of blackberries has about 7–8 grams of fiber—that's over 25% of your daily needs.

- Promotes regular bowel movements, feeds healthy gut bacteria, and may reduce the risk of colon cancer.

## 5. Supports Immune Function

- Loaded with **vitamin C** (one serving gives you 30 %+ of your daily value).

- Vitamin C boosts immune cell function and helps your body heal from wounds and illness faster.

## 6. May Help Fight Cancer

- Compounds like ellagic acid, quercetin, and anthocyanins have anti-cancer properties.

- These may slow tumor growth and help your body detox potential carcinogens.

### 7. Good for Bones and Skin

- Contains vitamin K and manganese—essential for bone strength, wound healing, and collagen formation.

- The vitamin C content also supports skin elasticity and collagen production, keeping your skin firm and youthful.

### 8. Supports Blood Sugar Balance

- Despite being sweet, blackberries have a low glycemic index and are high in fiber.

- They may help improve insulin sensitivity and keep blood sugar levels stable—great for people with diabetes or prediabetes.

### 9. Oral Health

- Blackberries have natural antibacterial properties that may help fight oral bacteria, reduce gum inflammation, and support healthy teeth and gums.

## Chia Seeds

I put chia seeds into my daily smoothie. It makes it thicker when blended with my magic mixture. Here are some benefits of chia seeds:

**Fiber**: Chia seeds are an excellent source of soluble fiber, which helps with digestion, supports gut health, and promotes feelings of fullness.

**Omega-3 Fatty Acids**: They are rich in alpha-linolenic acid (ALA), a type of plant-based omega-3 fatty acid that supports heart health and reduces inflammation.

1. **Protein:** Chia seeds are a good plant-based protein source, making them great for vegetarians and vegans.

2. **Vitamins and Minerals:** Chia seeds are high in calcium, magnesium, phosphorus, and manganese, which support bone health, energy production, and metabolic function.

3. **Antioxidants:** These seeds contain antioxidants, such as flavonoids and polyphenols, which help protect cells from oxidative damage.

4. **Lowers Cholesterol:** The high omega-3 content in chia seeds helps reduce LDL (bad) cholesterol and improve overall cholesterol levels, contributing to heart health.

5. **Reduces Inflammation:** Omega-3s in chia seeds are also known to reduce inflammation, which can lower the risk of chronic diseases like heart disease.

6. **Blood Pressure:** Some studies suggest that chia seeds may help lower blood pressure, particularly in people with high blood pressure.

7. **High in Calcium:** Chia seeds are an excellent plant-based source of calcium, essential for maintaining strong bones and teeth.

## Flax Meal

I've always known that flax seeds or flaxseed oil is good for my hair and skin. People comment on how great my skin looks all the time. I guess putting flax meal in my smoothie every day helps. I do notice thicker hair around my edges these days. Let's get a further breakdown of the magic found in flax meal, and perhaps you'll want to use it too.

1. **Alpha-Linolenic Acid (ALA)**: Flax meal is one of the best plant-based sources of omega-3 fatty acids, specifically ALA, which helps reduce inflammation, improve heart health, and support brain function.

2. **Heart Health**: The omega-3s in flax meal have been shown to lower bad cholesterol (LDL), reduce inflammation, and improve overall cardiovascular health. This can reduce the risk of heart disease, stroke, and other cardiovascular conditions.

3. **Soluble Fiber**: Flax meal is high in soluble fiber, which helps with digestion and can slow down the absorption of sugars in the bloodstream. This can help stabilize blood sugar levels and support a healthy weight.

4. **Insoluble Fiber**: It also contains insoluble fiber, which adds bulk to stool and promotes regular bowel movements, helping to prevent constipation and support gut health.

5. **Gut Health**: The fiber in flax meal acts as a prebiotic, promoting the growth of beneficial bacteria in the gut, improving digestion, and boosting overall gut health.

6. **Omega-3s for Cognitive Health**: The ALA in flax meal is beneficial for cognitive function and brain health. Omega-3 fatty acids are known to improve memory, mood, and cognitive performance.

7. **Mental Clarity**: Regular consumption of flax meal can help enhance mental clarity, focus, and may help reduce the risk of neurodegenerative conditions like Alzheimer's.

8. **Lowering Cholesterol**: Flax meal is rich in lignans and fiber, which can help lower blood cholesterol levels by improving lipid profiles, reducing triglycerides, and increasing **good cholesterol** (HDL).

9. **Blood Pressure**: The omega-3 fatty acids in flax meal also help **lower blood pressure**, which is another key factor in maintaining heart health.

10. **Reduces Inflammation**: Flax meal's omega-3 content has anti-inflammatory properties that help reduce overall inflammation in the body, which is important for heart disease prevention.

## Sunflower Lecithin

When I got wind that I needed to get my cholesterol under control, I immediately sought out a natural solution. My nutritional buddy Asabi recommended lecithin. Not being a pill-taker, I first got liquid lecithin. Lawdy Lawd, it was mega thick and stuck to the sides of anything it touched. To thin it out, I mixed it with a little coconut oil. Once I used up the liquid, I purchased a Sunflower lecithin powder. This works well in my smoothie and takes away the messiness I experienced with using the thick liquid version. Here are some of the benefits of sunflower lecithin:

1. **Protects Brain Cells**: The choline found in sunflower lecithin helps maintain the integrity of cell membranes, particularly in the brain, supporting neural communication and brain health.

2. **Lowers Cholesterol**: Sunflower lecithin may help lower LDL (bad) cholesterol levels and increase HDL (good) cholesterol, promoting better cardiovascular health.

3. **Liver Health:** Phosphatidylcholine in lecithin supports liver function and can help prevent fat accumulation in the liver, reducing the risk of fatty liver disease.

4. **Anti-inflammatory**: The healthy fats in sunflower lecithin have anti-inflammatory effects, which can support overall cardiovascular health and help reduce the risk of heart disease.

## Nutritional Yeast

Nutritional Yeast is a staple food in my home. I take it to help manage my sugar and neurological health. Here are some of its benefits:

1. **B Vitamins**: It's especially high in B vitamins, including B12 (if fortified), B6, thiamine (B1), riboflavin (B2), and folate. B vitamins are crucial for energy production, brain health, and maintaining a healthy nervous system. B vitamins, especially B12, play a key role in brain health. They are essential for producing neurotransmitters.

2. **Minerals:** It provides zinc, selenium, and iron, which are important for immune function, antioxidant protection, and overall health.

3. **May Help Prevent Cognitive Decline**: Some studies suggest that B12, which is often lacking in vegan diets, can help prevent memory loss and other cognitive issues, particularly in older adults.

4. **Mood Boost**: Adequate levels of B6 and B12 can help regulate mood and reduce symptoms of anxiety or depression, which are often linked to deficiencies in these vitamins.

5. **Protein:** Nutritional yeast is a good source of complete protein, containing all nine essential amino acids, making it an excellent option for vegetarians and vegans.

6. **Cholesterol Management**: Nutritional yeast contains beta-glucans, a type of soluble fiber that has been shown to help lower cholesterol levels, which can reduce the risk of heart disease.

7. **Antioxidants**: Nutritional yeast is rich in antioxidants like glutathione and selenium, which help protect the cardiovascular system from oxidative stress and inflammation, both of which are risk factors for heart disease.

8. **Amino Acids**: The amino acids in nutritional yeast help support muscle function and tissue repair, contributing to overall heart health.

9. **Fortified B12**: Since **vitamin B12** is mostly found in animal products, **fortified nutritional yeast** is a great source of this important nutrient for those following a plant-based diet.

10. **Complete Protein**: As a plant-based complete protein, nutritional yeast is a great protein source for people who don't eat meat, helping support muscle maintenance and repair.

11. **Heart health** - The fiber in nutritional yeast, beta-glucan, may reduce cholesterol levels. Nutritional yeast is also a low-glycemic food that contains chromium, a mineral that may help regulate your blood sugar. Maintaining good blood sugar and cholesterol levels lowers your risk for diabetes and heart disease.

## Ceylon Cinnamon

I've always had a good experience taking cinnamon to manage my sugar. I learned that CEYLON cinnamon was the type of cinnamon I should have been using. The first cinnamon I used burned like crazy when I put it under my tongue. I was surprised to see that the Ceylon cinnamon did not burn. Now I keep large quantities on deck in my kitchen and use a tablespoon in my smoothie. Here are some of Cylon's benefits:

1. **Improves insulin sensitivity**: Ceylon cinnamon helps the body use insulin more effectively, which can lead to better blood sugar control.

2. **Lowers fasting blood glucose**: Studies have shown that it may help reduce fasting blood sugar levels, especially in individuals with type 2 diabetes or insulin resistance.

3. **Slows carbohydrate digestion**: It may slow the breakdown of carbohydrates in the digestive tract, reducing post-meal blood sugar spikes.

4. **Lowers cholesterol and triglycerides**: Ceylon cinnamon may reduce **LDL (bad cholesterol)** and **triglycerides** while increasing **HDL (good cholesterol)**.

5. **Anti-inflammatory effects**: It helps reduce chronic inflammation, a known contributor to heart disease and other metabolic conditions.

6. **Improves blood flow**: Cinnamon may help relax blood vessels and improve circulation, which can help regulate blood pressure.

7. **May lower hypertension risk**: Early studies suggest it can help reduce elevated blood pressure levels in some individuals.

## HERE ARE SOME GREAT RECIPES FOR MY DAILY SALAD

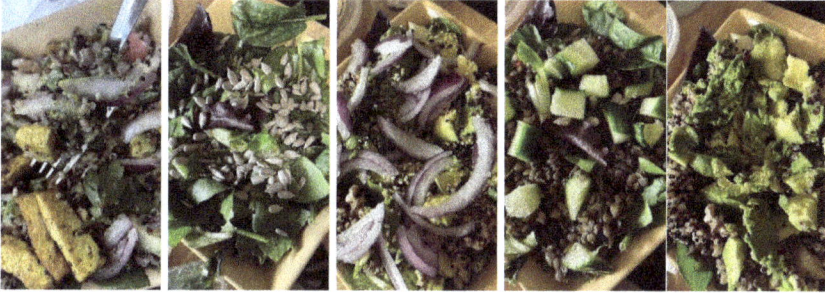

After my celery juice and smoothie in the morning, I break out the goods for my daily salad! This lovely combo fills me up for the day. My salads are nothing short of SLAYTASTIC! Check out the ingredients below and the benefits of everything I put into my SUPER SALAD.

### Baby Spinach

### 1. Brain & Nervous System Support

- Rich in folate **(vitamin B9)**, which supports brain function, mood regulation, and healthy neural development, especially important during pregnancy.

- **Vitamin K** and **nitrates** in spinach may also improve blood flow to the brain and help protect against age-related cognitive decline.

### 2. Heart Health

- High in nitrates, which help relax blood vessels, lower blood pressure, and improve circulation.

- Contains potassium, magnesium, and fiber, all of which help regulate blood pressure and cholesterol.

## 3. Rich in Iron

- Spinach contains non-heme iron, important for red blood cell production and preventing **fatigue** and anemia.

- Pair it with vitamin C–rich foods (like strawberries or lemon juice) to enhance iron absorption.

## 4. Supports Bone Strength

- Loaded with **vitamin K1**, which helps with calcium regulation and strengthens bones.

- Also contains small amounts of **calcium**, **magnesium**, and **phosphorus**—key minerals for bone health.

## 5. Antioxidant Protection

- Packed with antioxidants like lutein, zeaxanthin, beta-carotene, and vitamin C, which protect cells from free radical damage.

- These compounds may help reduce the risk of chronic diseases like cancer, diabetes, and heart disease.

## 6. Eye Health

- Contains lutein and zeaxanthin, two carotenoids that accumulate in the retina and help prevent macular degeneration and cataracts.

## 7. Anti-Inflammatory Effects

- The antioxidants and polyphenols in spinach help reduce systemic inflammation, which plays a role in nearly every chronic disease.

## 8. Supports Digestive Health

- A good source of fiber, which helps:
  - Regulate bowel movements
  - Feed beneficial gut bacteria
  - Support detox and healthy digestion

## 9. Great for Pregnancy

- High in folate, which is critical for fetal neural tube development.

- Also provides iron, calcium, and vitamin A, which are key nutrients during pregnancy.

### Spring Mix Salad

## 1. Nutrient-Dense & Low in Calories:

- Spring mix is low in calories but high in essential nutrients like:
  - Vitamin A
  - Vitamin C
  - Vitamin K
  - Folate
  - Iron

- o Calcium
- You get a wide variety of micronutrients in just a small serving.

## 2. Heart-Healthy

- Rich in fiber, potassium, and antioxidants, all of which help:
  - o Lower blood pressure
  - o Improve cholesterol levels
  - o Reduce inflammation in blood vessels
- Greens like arugula and spinach contain nitrates that improve blood flow and circulation.

## 3. Brain & Mood Support

- Folate (B9) supports brain development and mental clarity.
- Vitamin K plays a role in brain cell signaling and may help protect against cognitive decline.

## 4. Eye Health

- Greens like spinach, kale, and romaine are rich in lutein and zeaxanthin, two carotenoids that protect against macular degeneration and blue light damage.

## 5. Supports Bone Health

- High in vitamin K, calcium, and magnesium, which all contribute to bone strength and mineralization.
- Vitamin K is especially important for calcium absorption and preventing bone loss.

## 6. Boosts Digestive Health

- Good source of dietary fiber, which:
    - Supports healthy gut bacteria
    - Promotes regular digestion
    - Keeps you feeling full longer (helps with weight management)

## 7. Antioxidant Powerhouse

- Every green in the mix has its own set of polyphenols, flavonoids, and phytonutrients.
- Together, they help combat oxidative stress, lower inflammation, and may reduce the risk of chronic disease.

## 8. Hydrating and Alkalizing

- Leafy greens are high in water content, helping keep you hydrated.
- They also alkalize, which may support pH balance and reduce acid load in the body.

## 9. Excellent for Pregnancy

- Folate, iron, calcium, and vitamin A in spring mix support fetal development and maternal health.

## Cucumber

Growing up, I never liked cucumbers. As I continued to read up on things like food combining and food needed based on your body type, I found that cucumbers were exactly what I needed to eat. The facts below prove my point. Here are some cucumber benefits:

1. **Hydration:** Cucumbers are made up of about 95% water, making them excellent for hydration and maintaining proper fluid balance in the body.

2. **Rich in Nutrients**: Cucumbers provide vitamins and minerals like vitamin K, vitamin C, potassium, and magnesium, which are important for overall health.

3. **Antioxidant Properties**: They contain antioxidants like beta-carotene and flavonoids, which help neutralize free radicals and reduce oxidative stress in the body.

4. **Supports Skin Health:** Cucumbers are great for your skin. The high-water content helps to keep your skin hydrated, and cucumbers have compounds that reduce swelling and irritation, making them a common ingredient in skincare products.

5. **Aid in Digestion**: The fiber in cucumbers, particularly in the peel, promotes healthy digestion by supporting regular bowel movements and preventing constipation.

6. **Weight Management**: With their low calorie and high-water content, cucumbers are great for those looking to maintain or lose weight, as they provide a feeling of fullness with minimal calories.

7. **Promotes Heart Health**: Cucumbers are a good source of potassium, which helps lower blood pressure and supports

cardiovascular health by maintaining healthy blood circulation.

8. **Anti-Inflammatory**: Cucumbers contain compounds that have anti-inflammatory properties, which can help in reducing swelling and pain, especially in conditions like arthritis.

9. **Detoxification**: Cucumbers help in flushing out toxins from the body due to their high water content, supporting kidney and liver function.

10. **Improves Bone Health**: The vitamin K content in cucumbers is important for bone health as it plays a vital role in calcium absorption and bone mineralization.

## Garlic

Who cares about garlic breath when it does so many good things for the body? I even used fresh garlic when I was in Africa, to ward away mosquitoes. They don't like the taste of garlic in your blood…just like Dracula! Here are some benefits of adding garlic to your diet:

1. **Boosts Immune System**: Garlic has natural antibacterial, antiviral, and antifungal properties. It can help strengthen the immune system and reduce the risk of infections by enhancing the body's ability to fight off harmful pathogens.

2. **Heart Health:** Garlic has been shown to help reduce blood pressure, lower cholesterol levels, and improve overall heart health. It can help lower the risk of heart disease by reducing bad cholesterol (LDL) and preventing the formation of blood clots.

3. **Rich in Antioxidants**: Garlic contains powerful antioxidants, such as allicin, which help fight oxidative stress in the body. This can help reduce inflammation and lower the risk of chronic diseases like cancer and diabetes.

4. **Anti-Inflammatory Effects**: The compounds in garlic, especially allicin, have anti-inflammatory properties that can help reduce chronic inflammation, which is linked to various health conditions, including arthritis.

5. **Supports Digestive Health**: Garlic can improve digestion by stimulating the production of digestive enzymes and supporting the health of the gut. It may also help in preventing issues like bloating and indigestion.

6. **Detoxification:** Garlic contains sulfur compounds that help detoxify the body by promoting the elimination of toxins. It can support the liver in detoxifying harmful substances and promote overall detox health.

7. **Improves Bone Health**: Some studies suggest that garlic may improve bone health by increasing estrogen levels in women, which may help reduce the risk of osteoporosis and promote stronger bones.

8. **Enhances Brain Health**: The antioxidants in garlic help protect brain cells from oxidative stress, which may help reduce the risk of cognitive decline and neurodegenerative diseases like Alzheimer's.

9. **Helps Regulate Blood Sugar Levels**: Garlic has been found to improve insulin sensitivity, which can be helpful for those

with type 2 diabetes or those trying to regulate their blood sugar levels.

10. **Supports Respiratory Health**: Garlic has been traditionally used to treat respiratory issues such as colds, coughs, and asthma. Its antimicrobial properties can help clear up respiratory infections and support overall lung health.

11. **Anti-Cancer Properties**: Some studies have suggested that the compounds in garlic may help slow down the growth of cancer cells, particularly in cancers of the stomach, colon, and esophagus. Antioxidants in garlic also help protect cells from DNA damage.

12. **Promotes Healthy Skin**: The antimicrobial and anti-inflammatory properties of garlic can help with skin conditions such as acne, eczema, and fungal infections. It also supports the healing of wounds.

Garlic can be eaten raw or cooked, and while cooking it may reduce some of its medicinal properties, it still retains a good amount of health benefits. For optimal benefits, it's often recommended to crush or chop garlic and let it sit for a few minutes before eating to activate its active compounds like allicin.

## Quinoa

I love quinoa! I started eating it when I stopped eating rice. It doesn't have the same texture as rice, yet it is a good complement to veggies in my salad and to cooked veggies too. Quinoa is often referred to as a "superfood" due to its impressive nutritional profile and numerous health benefits. Here are some key benefits of quinoa:

1. **High in Protein**: Quinoa is a complete protein, meaning it contains all nine essential amino acids that the body cannot produce on its own. This makes it an excellent plant-based protein source, especially for vegetarians and vegans.

2. **Rich in Fiber**: Quinoa is a great source of dietary fiber, which aids in digestion and helps prevent constipation. It also promotes feelings of fullness, which can aid in weight management by preventing overeating.

3. **Gluten-Free**: Quinoa is naturally gluten-free, making it a great option for people with celiac disease or gluten sensitivity. It can be used as a gluten-free substitute for grains like wheat, barley, and rye.

4. **Packed with Nutrients**: Quinoa is rich in vitamins and minerals, including magnesium, manganese, phosphorus, folate, iron, and B-vitamins. These nutrients support overall health, including bone health, energy production, and immune function.

5. **Supports Heart Health**: The high fiber content in quinoa helps lower cholesterol levels, and its healthy fats (particularly unsaturated fats) may help reduce the risk of heart disease. Quinoa also contains antioxidants that help fight inflammation, another risk factor for heart disease.

6. **Regulates Blood Sugar Levels**: Quinoa has a low glycemic index, meaning it has a smaller impact on blood sugar levels

compared to other grains. This makes it a good option for people with diabetes or those looking to maintain stable energy levels throughout the day.

7. **Aids in Weight Management**: Due to its high protein and fiber content, quinoa can help promote feelings of fullness, reduce appetite, and prevent overeating. It can also stabilize blood sugar levels, helping to prevent insulin spikes and crashes that contribute to hunger.

8. **High in Antioxidants**: Quinoa is rich in antioxidants, including flavonoids like quercetin and kaempferol. These antioxidants help fight oxidative stress and inflammation in the body, which may reduce the risk of chronic diseases, including cancer and neurodegenerative conditions.

9. **Supports Bone Health**: Quinoa contains significant amounts of magnesium, manganese, and phosphorus, all of which are essential for maintaining strong, healthy bones. This makes quinoa a good addition to a diet for bone health.

10. **Good for Digestive Health**: The fiber in quinoa supports gut health by promoting regular bowel movements and nourishing beneficial gut bacteria. It can also reduce the risk of digestive disorders like irritable bowel syndrome (IBS).

11. **Easy to Digest**: Unlike some other grains, quinoa is generally easier to digest. It's often recommended for people with digestive issues or for those who have trouble digesting wheat or other grains.

12. **Versatile in Cooking**: Quinoa is easy to cook and can be used in a variety of dishes, such as salads, soups, stir-fries, and even as a breakfast cereal. Its mild, nutty flavor makes it a versatile alternative to rice, couscous, or pasta.

## Red Onions

Turns out the red onions are better for you than any others. They seem to have more antioxidants. I personally love the "color pop" they give my food. Here are some key benefits of red onions:

1. **Rich in Antioxidants**: Red onions are packed with antioxidants, particularly anthocyanins, which give them their deep purple-red color. These antioxidants help combat oxidative stress, reducing the risk of chronic diseases like heart disease, cancer, and diabetes.

2. **Supports Heart Health**: Red onions have been shown to help improve cardiovascular health by reducing cholesterol levels, lowering blood pressure, and preventing blood clots. The antioxidants and sulfur compounds in red onions can help reduce inflammation, which is a key factor in heart disease.

3. **Anti-Inflammatory Properties**: Red onions contain quercetin, a powerful antioxidant that has anti-inflammatory effects. This can help reduce inflammation in the body, which is linked to various chronic conditions, such as arthritis and asthma.

4. **Improves Digestion**: Red onions are a good source of dietary fiber, which helps promote healthy digestion by supporting

regular bowel movements. The fiber also feeds beneficial gut bacteria, which are essential for a healthy digestive system.

5. **Supports Immune System**: Red onions are rich in vitamin C, which is essential for a strong immune system. Vitamin C helps fight infections, supports the production of white blood cells, and acts as an antioxidant to protect the body from harmful pathogens.

6. **Blood Sugar Regulation**: The sulfur compounds and quercetin in red onions may help regulate blood sugar levels by improving insulin sensitivity. This can be beneficial for those with type 2 diabetes or those looking to maintain stable blood sugar levels.

7. **Cancer Prevention**: Some studies suggest that the compounds found in red onions, including quercetin and sulfur compounds, may help reduce the growth of cancer cells. They have been shown to inhibit the spread of cancer cells in certain types of cancers, including colon, breast, and stomach cancers.

8. **Improves Skin Health**: The antioxidants in red onions, especially vitamin C and quercetin, can help protect the skin from damage caused by free radicals. Red onions may also help with conditions like acne due to their antibacterial properties.

9. **Supports Bone Health**: Red onions contain nutrients such as calcium, phosphorus, and magnesium, which contribute to bone health. Some studies have shown that regular

consumption of onions may help increase bone density and reduce the risk of osteoporosis.

10. **Detoxifying Properties**: Red onions have natural detoxifying properties, helping to cleanse the body of harmful toxins. Their sulfur compounds may promote liver health and help eliminate toxins more efficiently.

11. **Helps with Hair Health**: The sulfur compounds in red onions are thought to promote healthy hair growth. Some people use onion juice as a home remedy to improve hair thickness and reduce hair loss.

12. **Natural Antibacterial and Antifungal:** Red onions have natural antibacterial and antifungal properties, which can help protect the body from infections. They can be particularly helpful in preventing skin infections and supporting overall immune health.

## Walnuts

I was craving walnuts one day and couldn't figure out why. So, if you know me, I went to look up how walnuts benefit the body. Right away, I learned that they were good food for sugar maintenance. So that's what the craving was about, I saw. With the development of this book, I've found out so many more reasons as to why walnuts belong in my body daily. Walnuts are a nutrient-dense food that offers numerous health benefits. Here are some of the key benefits of incorporating walnuts into your diet:

1. **Rich in Healthy Fats**: Walnuts are an excellent source of healthy fats, especially omega-3 fatty acids (in the form of alpha-linolenic acid, or ALA), which are essential for brain function, heart health, and reducing inflammation in the body.

2. **Supports Heart Health**: The omega-3 fatty acids, antioxidants, and healthy fats in walnuts help lower bad cholesterol (LDL), reduce inflammation, and improve overall heart health. Consuming walnuts regularly can reduce the risk of heart disease and stroke.

3. **Brain Health and Cognitive Function**: Walnuts are known for their positive effects on brain health. The omega-3 fatty acids, polyphenols, and antioxidants in walnuts may improve cognitive function, memory, and even help protect against age-related mental decline and neurodegenerative diseases like Alzheimer's.

4. **Anti-Inflammatory Effects**: Walnuts contain polyphenolic compounds that have anti-inflammatory properties. These compounds help reduce chronic inflammation, which is linked to various health issues, including arthritis, heart disease, and diabetes.

5. **Improves Gut Health**: The fiber content in walnuts supports digestive health by promoting regular bowel movements and nourishing beneficial gut bacteria. A healthy gut microbiome is crucial for overall health and immune function.

6. **Helps Control Weight**: Despite being calorie-dense, walnuts can help with weight management. The combination of healthy fats, protein, and fiber in walnuts helps promote

satiety (feeling of fullness), reducing the likelihood of overeating.

7. **Rich in Antioxidants**: Walnuts contain powerful antioxidants, such as vitamin E and polyphenols, which help neutralize harmful free radicals in the body. This helps reduce oxidative stress and may lower the risk of chronic diseases like cancer.

8. **Blood Sugar Regulation**: Walnuts may help regulate blood sugar levels due to their healthy fat, fiber, and protein content. This can be beneficial for people with type 2 diabetes or those looking to maintain stable blood sugar levels.

9. **Supports Bone Health**: Walnuts provide essential minerals like magnesium, phosphorus, and calcium, which are important for maintaining strong bones. Regular walnut consumption may help reduce the risk of bone-related conditions, such as osteoporosis.

10. **Promotes Healthy Skin**: The antioxidants and healthy fats in walnuts can help protect the skin from oxidative damage caused by environmental factors like UV rays and pollution. The anti-inflammatory properties of walnuts may also help reduce conditions like acne or eczema.

11. **Improves Mood and Reduces Stress**: Walnuts contain magnesium and other nutrients that may help reduce stress, improve mood, and support mental well-being. Some studies suggest that regular walnut consumption may be linked to a lower risk of depression and anxiety.

12. **Improves Sleep Quality**: Walnuts contain melatonin, a hormone that helps regulate sleep. Including walnuts in your diet may improve sleep quality and help with insomnia or irregular sleep patterns.

Incorporating walnuts into your daily diet is easy—they can be eaten on their own as a snack, added to salads, mixed into smoothies, or used in baked goods. Just a small handful (about 1 ounce or 28 grams) per day can provide significant health benefits!

## Apples

"Cosmic apples" refer to a variety of apples known as Cosmic Crisp apples, which were developed by Washington State University and are a cross between the "Honeycrisp" and "Enterprise" apple varieties. They are known for their crisp texture, sweetness, and long shelf life. Like other apple varieties, Cosmic Crisp apples offer several health benefits, thanks to their rich nutritional content. Here are some of the key benefits of Cosmic apples:

### 1. Rich in Nutrients

Cosmic apples are packed with essential nutrients, including:

- **Fiber:** One medium-sized apple provides about 4 grams of dietary fiber, which is important for digestion and helps keep you feeling full.

- **Vitamins**: Cosmic apples are a good source of vitamin C, which is vital for immune health, skin health, and reducing oxidative stress.

- **Antioxidants**: Cosmic apples are rich in antioxidants, particularly flavonoids and polyphenols, which help fight free radicals and inflammation in the body.

## 2. Supports Heart Health

- **Lower Cholesterol**: The fiber in Cosmic apples, especially pectin, can help lower bad cholesterol (LDL) levels, contributing to better heart health.

- **Blood Pressure Regulation**: The potassium content in apples can help regulate blood pressure, reducing the risk of heart disease and stroke.

## 3. Aids in Digestion

- The fiber in Cosmic apples promotes healthy digestion by supporting regular bowel movements and preventing constipation. The soluble fiber in apples can also help maintain a healthy gut microbiome.

## 4. Helps with Weight Management

- Cosmic apples are low in calories but high in fiber and water content, which can help keep you full and satisfied for longer. This can reduce overall calorie intake and help with weight management.

## 5. Supports Immune Function

- The vitamin C content in Cosmic apples boosts the immune system by promoting the production of white blood cells, which help the body fight infections and illnesses.

## 6. Regulates Blood Sugar Levels

- The fiber and natural sugars in apples are released slowly into the bloodstream, which helps prevent blood sugar spikes. This makes Cosmic apples a good option for people with diabetes or those looking to maintain stable blood sugar levels.

## 7. Promotes Healthy Skin

- The antioxidants, vitamin C, and water content in Cosmic apples contribute to healthy, glowing skin by protecting it from oxidative damage and helping maintain moisture levels.

## 8. Improves Oral Health

- Eating apples, including Cosmic apples, can help promote oral health. The crunchy texture helps stimulate the production of saliva, which neutralizes acids in the mouth and prevents tooth decay. The natural compounds in apples may also help reduce the growth of harmful bacteria in the mouth.

## 9. Protects Against Chronic Diseases

- The antioxidants and phytochemicals in apples are associated with a reduced risk of chronic diseases, including certain types of cancer, heart disease, and neurodegenerative diseases like Alzheimer's.

## 10. Boosts Mental Health

- Apples, including Cosmic apples, contain certain nutrients that may have a positive effect on mental well-being. The flavonoids and antioxidants in apples may help reduce inflammation in the brain, improving mood and cognitive function.

## 11. Hydrating and Refreshing

- Cosmic apples have a high water content, making them a hydrating and refreshing snack, especially on hot days. Staying hydrated is important for overall health, and apples can be a delicious way to support hydration.

## 12. Promotes Healthy Vision

- Apples contain small amounts of vitamin A and other antioxidants, which can help maintain eye health and reduce the risk of age-related vision problems like macular degeneration.

## Sunflower Seeds

When I got a sense of the benefits of sunflower seeds, I made a decision to simply sprinkle them over my salads regularly. Just from an aesthetic standpoint, I love the texture the seeds add to my salad. Here are some of the key benefits of sunflower seeds:

## 1. Rich in Nutrients

- **Vitamin E**: Sunflower seeds are particularly rich in vitamin E, an antioxidant that helps protect cells from oxidative stress and supports skin health.

- **Magnesium**: They provide a good amount of magnesium, which is important for muscle and nerve function, as well as bone health.

- **Selenium:** Sunflower seeds contain selenium, an important mineral that helps protect the body from oxidative damage and supports thyroid function.

- **B Vitamins**: Sunflower seeds are a good source of B vitamins like folate, niacin, and vitamin B6, which help with energy production and support the nervous system.

## 2. Supports Heart Health

- **Healthy Fats**: Sunflower seeds are high in polyunsaturated fats, including omega-6 fatty acids, which are important for heart health. These healthy fats can help reduce bad cholesterol (LDL) and lower the risk of heart disease.

- **Antioxidants**: The vitamin E and other antioxidants in sunflower seeds help reduce inflammation and oxidative stress, both of which are linked to heart disease.

- **Cholesterol Regulation**: Studies suggest that sunflower seeds can help lower cholesterol levels, making them a heart-healthy snack.

## 3. Promotes Healthy Skin

- **Rich in Vitamin E**: Vitamin E is known for its skin-protective properties. It helps prevent skin aging, protects against UV damage, and supports the healing of skin wounds.

- **Anti-Inflammatory**: Sunflower seeds have anti-inflammatory properties, which can benefit skin conditions like acne or eczema.

## 4. Supports Immune Function

- **Antioxidants and Minerals**: The vitamin E, selenium, and zinc in sunflower seeds boost immune function by protecting cells from free radical damage and supporting the production of white blood cells, which help fight infections.

- **Anti-Inflammatory Effects**: The anti-inflammatory compounds in sunflower seeds help to strengthen the immune system and reduce inflammation in the body.

## 5. Improves Digestion

- High in Fiber: Sunflower seeds are a good source of dietary fiber, which supports healthy digestion and regular bowel movements. Fiber also feeds beneficial gut bacteria, promoting a healthy gut microbiome.

- **Gut Health**: The fiber content can help prevent constipation and promote overall digestive health.

## 6. Aids in Weight Management

- **High Protein and Fiber**: Sunflower seeds are high in both protein and fiber, which can help increase feelings of fullness and reduce overall calorie intake. Including them as a snack can help control hunger and prevent overeating.

- **Healthy Fats**: The healthy fats in sunflower seeds help keep you satisfied, making them a good option for controlling appetite.

## 7. Blood Sugar Control

- **Supports Insulin Sensitivity**: Some studies suggest that sunflower seeds can help improve insulin sensitivity, making them beneficial for managing blood sugar levels, especially for people with type 2 diabetes.

- **Low Glycemic Index**: Sunflower seeds have a low glycemic index, meaning they have a minimal impact on blood sugar levels compared to high-glycemic foods.

## 8. Supports Bone Health

- **Magnesium and Phosphorus**: Sunflower seeds contain magnesium and phosphorus, both of which are important for maintaining strong and healthy bones. They help in calcium absorption and bone mineralization.

## 9. Improves Mood and Reduces Stress

- **Magnesium**: Sunflower seeds are a good source of magnesium, which has been linked to improved mood and relaxation. Magnesium helps regulate the production of neurotransmitters that control mood and stress levels.

- **Serotonin Production**: The amino acid **tryptophan** in sunflower seeds helps in the production of serotonin, a neurotransmitter that regulates mood and promotes feelings of happiness.

## 10. Supports Hair Health

- **Zinc and Vitamin E**: Zinc and vitamin E in sunflower seeds help promote healthy hair growth and improve the condition of the scalp. Zinc also supports the production of hair follicles, while vitamin E supports circulation to the scalp.

## 11. Promotes Brain Health

- **Healthy Fats and Antioxidants**: The omega-6 fatty acids, antioxidants, and vitamin E in sunflower seeds are beneficial for brain health. They help reduce inflammation in the brain and support cognitive function, potentially reducing the risk of neurodegenerative diseases like Alzheimer's.

## 12. Bone Health

- The magnesium and phosphorus in sunflower seeds work together to support bone strength and health, contributing to proper bone formation and mineralization.

## Lentils

My, my, my, I just love me some lentils. I've always loved them as a soup, and now I love them all over my salad too. I love yellow lentils and pink ones. Lately, though, the brown lentils suit me just fine. They are packed with protein, fiber, vitamins, and minerals. Here are some of the key benefits of lentils:

## 1. High in Plant-Based Protein

Lentils are an excellent source of plant-based protein, making them a great option for vegetarians and vegans. They provide essential amino acids, which are important for muscle growth, tissue repair, and overall bodily functions. One cup of cooked lentils provides around 18 grams of protein.

## 2. Rich in Dietary Fiber

Lentils are high in fiber, which is beneficial for digestive health. Fiber helps promote regular bowel movements, prevents constipation, and supports a healthy gut microbiome. It also helps reduce the risk of digestive disorders like diverticulosis and irritable bowel syndrome (IBS).

## 3. Supports Heart Health

- **Cholesterol Reduction**: The soluble fiber in lentils can help reduce levels of LDL (bad) cholesterol, which is a major risk factor for heart disease.

- **Blood Pressure Regulation**: Lentils are rich in potassium and magnesium, both of which help regulate blood pressure and support overall heart health.

- **Anti-Inflammatory Properties**: Lentils contain antioxidants, including flavonoids, which help reduce inflammation and lower the risk of chronic diseases, including cardiovascular diseases.

## 4. Helps Control Blood Sugar Levels

Lentils have a low glycemic index (GI), meaning they cause a slower, more gradual rise in blood sugar levels. This makes them an excellent choice for people with diabetes or those looking to stabilize their blood sugar levels. The fiber content also helps improve insulin sensitivity and blood glucose control.

## 5. Supports Weight Management

- **High in Fiber and Protein**: Lentils are low in calories but high in fiber and protein, which can help you feel full for longer, reducing overall calorie intake. This makes them a great addition to a weight-loss or weight-management plan.

- **Satiety**: The fiber and protein in lentils promote satiety, helping you avoid overeating or snacking between meals.

## 6. Rich in Essential Vitamins and Minerals

- **Iron**: Essential for the production of red blood cells and preventing anemia.

- **Folate**: Important for DNA synthesis and cell growth, and especially crucial for pregnant women to prevent neural tube defects in babies.

- **B Vitamins**: Lentils are rich in B-vitamins like B6, niacin, and pantothenic acid, which play important roles in energy production, brain function, and metabolism.

- **Magnesium**: Supports muscle and nerve function, bone health, and cardiovascular health.

- **Zinc**: Plays a role in immune function, wound healing, and DNA synthesis.

## 7. Supports Digestive Health

- **Gut Health**: The high fiber content in lentils helps promote the growth of beneficial bacteria in the gut, supporting a healthy microbiome. A healthy gut microbiome is important for immune function, digestion, and mental health.

- **Prevents Constipation**: Fiber in lentils helps prevent constipation by adding bulk to stool and promoting regular bowel movements.

## 8. Promotes Bone Health

Lentils contain minerals such as magnesium, phosphorus, and calcium, which are important for maintaining strong bones and preventing conditions like osteoporosis. The folate in lentils also plays a role in bone health by supporting the formation of bone-building cells.

## 9. Antioxidant-Rich

Lentils are packed with antioxidants such as polyphenols and flavonoids, which help combat oxidative stress and inflammation in the body. These antioxidants play a role in reducing the risk of chronic diseases, including heart disease, cancer, and neurodegenerative diseases like Alzheimer's.

## 10. Promotes Skin Health

The antioxidants, vitamins (especially B-vitamins), and minerals in lentils support healthy skin by protecting against oxidative damage. They may also help promote collagen production, which is essential for skin elasticity and reducing the appearance of wrinkles.

## 11. Mental Health

Lentils are a good source of folate, which has been linked to better mood regulation and a reduced risk of depression. Folate helps in the production of neurotransmitters like serotonin and dopamine, which are important for mood and mental well-being.

## Olive Tapenade

(Be aware of sodium content if watching blood pressure)

### 1.Rich in Healthy Fats

Olives and olive oil are known for their high content of monounsaturated fats, which are considered heart-healthy fats. These fats have been shown to:

- Help reduce bad cholesterol (LDL) levels while increasing good cholesterol (HDL), reducing the risk of heart disease.

- Support overall cardiovascular health by improving blood vessel function and reducing inflammation.

- Provide essential fatty acids that promote healthy brain function and hormone balance.

### 2. High in Antioxidants

Olives and olive oil are rich in antioxidants, including vitamin E, polyphenols, and oleuropein. These antioxidants help protect cells from oxidative damage caused by free radicals, which can reduce the risk of:

- Chronic diseases like heart disease, diabetes, and cancer.

- Premature aging and skin damage.

- Inflammation in the body, contributing to a reduced risk of inflammatory conditions.

### 3. Supports Digestive Health

The olives and olive oil in tapenade are rich in fiber, which aids in digestion and helps:

- Promote regular bowel movements.

- Improve gut health by feeding beneficial gut bacteria and supporting a healthy gut microbiome.

- Prevent constipation and support the overall digestive system.

### 4. Anti-Inflammatory Properties

Both olives and olive oil are known for their anti-inflammatory effects due to their high levels of polyphenols, such as oleocanthal. This can help:

- Reduce chronic inflammation, which is associated with conditions like arthritis, heart disease, and autoimmune disorders.

- Relieve pain and swelling related to inflammation, providing potential benefits for conditions like osteoarthritis.

### 5. Rich in Essential Nutrients

- **Vitamin E**: Supports immune function, skin health, and acts as a potent antioxidant.

- **Iron**: Important for oxygen transport and overall energy levels.

- **Copper**: Essential for the production of red blood cells and the maintenance of nerve and immune function.

- **Calcium**: Crucial for bone health and muscle function.

- **Magnesium**: Supports nerve function, muscle relaxation, and bone health.

## 6. Good for Skin Health

Olive oil is widely known for its skin benefits, thanks to its antioxidant properties and its ability to lock in moisture. Applying olive oil (or consuming it as part of a balanced diet) can help:

- Hydrate and protect the skin, reducing dryness and the appearance of wrinkles.

- Promote a glowing complexion and protect the skin from UV damage and pollution.

- Reduce inflammation and irritation in the skin, which may benefit conditions like eczema or acne.

## 7. Helps with Weight Management

Olive tapenade, when consumed in moderation, may support weight management. The healthy fats and fiber in the olives and olive oil help:

- Increase satiety, making you feel full for longer periods.

- Support fat metabolism, helping the body burn fat more efficiently.

- Keep hunger at bay, potentially reducing overall calorie intake.

## 8. May Improve Brain Health

The monounsaturated fats and **antioxidants** in olive oil have been shown to support brain health by:

- Reducing the risk of neurodegenerative diseases, such as Alzheimer's and Parkinson's.

- Improving cognitive function, memory, and learning abilities.

- Protecting the brain from oxidative damage and inflammation, which are linked to aging and mental decline.

## 9. Supports Bone Health

The polyphenols in olives and olive oil may help increase bone mineral density and protect against bone-related conditions such as osteoporosis. Consuming olive tapenade can support overall bone strength and help maintain a healthy skeletal system.

## 10. Supports Immune Health

Olive tapenade contains ingredients like garlic and capers, both of which have immune-boosting properties. Garlic is particularly known for:

- Helping the body fight infections by enhancing the immune response.

- Reducing the severity of colds and promoting general immune system health.

## Chickpeas

Chickpeas are also known as garbanzo beans. I love them! There are so many foods I love that are made from chickpeas. Hummus is huge on the list. Falafel is super loved and made of chickpeas, too. While all of this is good, I simply love the regular taste of chickpeas and adore them on my salad. I did notice they act as a starch in my system and can raise my sugar so I use them in moderation. Here are some of the key benefits of chickpeas:

### 1. High in Protein

Chickpeas are an excellent plant-based source of protein, making them a great choice for vegetarians, vegans, and those looking to reduce animal-based proteins. One cup of cooked chickpeas provides around 15 grams of protein. Protein is essential for:

- Muscle growth and repair.
- Supporting immune function.
- Maintaining healthy skin, hair, and nails.

### 2. Rich in Dietary Fiber

Chickpeas are high in fiber, which is beneficial for digestive health. **Fiber helps**:

- Promote regular bowel movements and prevent constipation.
- Feed beneficial gut bacteria, contributing to a healthy gut microbiome.

- Lower cholesterol levels, which can reduce the risk of heart disease.

- Control blood sugar levels, which is especially helpful for those with diabetes.

## 3. Supports Heart Health

Chickpeas support cardiovascular health in multiple ways:

- **Lower cholesterol**: The soluble fiber in chickpeas helps reduce levels of LDL (bad) cholesterol.

- **Blood pressure regulation**: Chickpeas are a good source of magnesium and potassium, which help maintain healthy blood pressure.

- **Anti-inflammatory**: The antioxidants and nutrients in chickpeas help reduce inflammation, lowering the risk of heart disease.

## 4. Helps Manage Blood Sugar Levels

Chickpeas have a low glycemic index (GI), meaning they cause a slower, more gradual rise in blood sugar levels. This makes them an excellent food choice for people with diabetes or those looking to maintain stable blood sugar. Additionally, the fiber and protein in chickpeas help improve insulin sensitivity and control blood sugar levels.

## 5. Supports Weight Management

- They are low in calories but high in protein and fiber, which help promote feelings of fullness and reduce overall calorie intake.

- The fiber content helps slow down digestion and keep you feeling satisfied for longer, reducing hunger cravings.

## 6. Packed with Essential Nutrients

Chickpeas provide a variety of important vitamins and minerals, including:

- **Folate (Vitamin B9)**: Crucial for DNA synthesis, cell growth, and development, especially important during pregnancy.

- **Iron**: Essential for transporting oxygen in the blood and preventing anemia.

- **Magnesium**: Supports muscle and nerve function and helps maintain bone health.

- **Phosphorus**: Important for healthy bones and teeth.

- **B Vitamins**: Help with energy production and maintaining healthy metabolism.

## 7. Promotes Digestive Health

The high fiber content in chickpeas supports digestive health by:

- **Improving gut health**: Fiber acts as a prebiotic, feeding the beneficial bacteria in the gut, which plays a role in overall health.

- **Preventing constipation**: Fiber helps bulk up stool and promotes regular bowel movements.

- **Reducing the risk of digestive disorders**, such as diverticulosis and inflammatory bowel diseases.

## 8. Good for Bone Health

Chickpeas contain several key nutrients that contribute to healthy bones, including:

- **Magnesium**: Supports bone mineralization and calcium absorption.
- **Calcium**: Crucial for strong bones and teeth.
- **Phosphorus**: Works with calcium to build and maintain healthy bones.

## 9. Improves Skin Health

Chickpeas are a good source of antioxidants, vitamins, and minerals that support skin health, including:

- **Vitamin A** and **Vitamin C**: Both are important for healthy, glowing skin and can help reduce signs of aging and skin damage.
- **Zinc**: Known for its role in reducing acne and promoting wound healing.

## 10. Anti-Inflammatory Benefits

Chickpeas contain compounds like polyphenols and saponins, which have anti-inflammatory properties. Chronic inflammation is linked to several diseases, including heart disease, diabetes, and arthritis, so consuming anti-inflammatory foods like chickpeas may help reduce the risk of these conditions.

## 11. Supports Immune Function

The vitamin C, iron, and zinc found in chickpeas help strengthen the immune system, allowing the body to fight infections and illnesses more effectively. Chickpeas also contain folate, which plays a role in immune health.

## 12. May Improve Mental Health

Some studies suggest that chickpeas may help improve mood and mental health due to their content of B vitamins (like folate and vitamin B6), which are involved in the production of neurotransmitters like serotonin and dopamine. These neurotransmitters are important for regulating mood and combating depression and anxiety.

## 13. Bone Health

Chickpeas contain calcium, magnesium, and phosphorus, which support the maintenance of strong bones and reduce the risk of conditions like osteoporosis.

## Apple Cider Vinegar

Folks complain about the flavor of Apple Cider Vinegar, but it doesn't bother me. I sprinkle it on my salad, and it adds great moisture to it. Apple cider vinegar (ACV) has gained popularity for its potential health benefits. Made from fermented apples, it contains acetic acid, which is thought to be responsible for many of its health-promoting properties. Here are some of the key benefits of apple cider vinegar:

## 1. Aids in Digestion

- **Improves Digestion**: ACV can help improve digestion by increasing stomach acid levels, which can aid in the breakdown of food and promote better nutrient absorption.

- **Soothes Acid Reflux**: Some people find that drinking a small amount of diluted apple cider vinegar can help alleviate symptoms of acid reflux or heartburn, as it can balance stomach acid levels.

- **Supports Healthy Gut Microbiome**: The acetic acid and probiotics in ACV help promote the growth of beneficial bacteria in the gut, which supports a healthy digestive system.

## 2. Supports Weight Loss

- **Appetite Suppression**: ACV has been shown to help reduce appetite by increasing feelings of fullness. The acetic acid may also slow down the digestion of starches, leading to less of an increase in blood sugar levels.

- **Boosts Metabolism**: Some studies suggest that apple cider vinegar can help increase metabolism, which may contribute to weight loss over time.

- **Helps Lower Blood Sugar**: ACV may improve insulin sensitivity and lower blood sugar levels after meals, which is beneficial for weight management and for people with diabetes.

### 3. Balances Blood Sugar Levels

- **Improves Insulin Sensitivity**: ACV has been shown to help lower blood sugar and improve insulin sensitivity, making it beneficial for those managing type 2 diabetes or prediabetes.

- **Regulates Blood Sugar After Meals**: Drinking diluted apple cider vinegar before or during meals may help lower post-meal blood sugar spikes, which is helpful for managing diabetes or even for those just looking to stabilize blood sugar levels.

### 4. Supports Heart Health

- **Lowers Cholesterol**: Some studies suggest that ACV may help reduce cholesterol levels by lowering total cholesterol and LDL (bad cholesterol), while increasing HDL (good cholesterol).

- **Reduces Blood Pressure**: ACV may have mild blood pressure-lowering effects, particularly for those with high blood pressure, due to its ability to promote a healthy balance of minerals like potassium and magnesium in the body.

### 5. Boosts Skin Health

- **Acne Treatment**: ACV has antibacterial and anti-inflammatory properties, making it useful in treating acne. It can be diluted with water and used as a toner to help balance the skin's pH and reduce the growth of acne-causing bacteria.

- **Soothes Sunburns**: ACV can be used in diluted form to help soothe sunburned skin, thanks to its anti-inflammatory properties.

- **Balances Skin pH**: The acidity of apple cider vinegar helps restore the natural pH of the skin, which can improve overall skin health.

## 6. Has Antimicrobial Properties

- **Fights Bacteria and Fungi**: The acetic acid in apple cider vinegar has antimicrobial properties, which can help kill harmful bacteria and fungi. It can be used to clean surfaces or treat minor cuts and scrapes.

- **Improves Oral Health**: Diluted ACV may help reduce bad breath by killing odor-causing bacteria in the mouth. It can also act as a mouthwash (though it should be used sparingly to avoid enamel erosion).

## 7. Detoxifies the Body

- **Liver Detox**: ACV is believed to help support liver detoxification by aiding in the removal of toxins from the body. It helps balance the body's pH and can improve liver function.

- **Promotes Lymphatic Drainage**: ACV is thought to promote better lymphatic drainage, which can help reduce swelling and support the body's natural detoxification process.

## 8. Helps with Bad Breath

- **Kills Odor-Causing Bacteria**: The acidic nature of ACV helps to kill the bacteria that can cause bad breath. Using diluted apple cider vinegar as a mouth rinse or gargling with it may help freshen your breath.

## 9. Improves Hair Health

- **Shiny Hair**: ACV can be used as a natural hair rinse to help restore shine, remove product buildup, and balance the scalp's pH. It may also help reduce dandruff by killing yeast and bacteria on the scalp.

- **Scalp Health**: ACV's antifungal and antibacterial properties can help keep your scalp healthy, reducing issues like dandruff or an itchy scalp.

## 10. Supports Immune Function

- **Boosts Immune System**: The probiotics and acetic acid in apple cider vinegar help promote a healthy gut microbiome, which is essential for immune system function. A balanced microbiome can improve the body's ability to fight infections and illnesses.

- **Rich in Antioxidants**: Apple cider vinegar contains antioxidants, including polyphenols, which can help reduce oxidative stress and support the immune system.

## 11. May Reduce Inflammation

- **Anti-inflammatory Effects**: Apple cider vinegar has anti-inflammatory properties that may help reduce symptoms of inflammatory conditions such as arthritis, joint pain, and muscle aches.

- **Alleviates Symptoms of Sore Throat**: Due to its antibacterial properties, gargling with diluted ACV may help soothe a sore throat and reduce inflammation in the throat.

## 12. May Improve Energy Levels

- **Balances pH and Electrolytes**: ACV helps balance the body's pH levels and provides a natural boost of energy. The potassium and enzymes in apple cider vinegar can also help replenish electrolytes, which can improve overall energy and hydration levels.

## Avocados

I have an avocado hack! Once your avocados are the consistency you want, put them in a jar of water and put that jar in the fridge. Those avocados that used to go bad before you could eat them will go bad no more! Putting them whole, with the skin intact, in that water, will keep them fresh for as long as an extra week or more. Try it for yourself and see! Thank me later!

Avocados are highly nutritious and offer a variety of health benefits due to their rich content of healthy fats, fiber, vitamins, and minerals. Here are some of the key benefits of avocados:

## 1. Rich in Healthy Fats

- **Monounsaturated Fats**: Avocados are an excellent source of heart-healthy monounsaturated fats, specifically oleic acid, which has been shown to reduce inflammation and may help lower the risk of heart disease.

- **Supports Cardiovascular Health**: The healthy fats in avocados help reduce bad cholesterol (LDL) and increase good cholesterol (HDL), promoting better cardiovascular health.

## 2. Nutrient-Dense

- **Vitamins**: Avocados are rich in vitamins such as vitamin K (important for bone health and blood clotting), vitamin E (an antioxidant that protects cells), vitamin C (supports the immune system and skin health), and several B-vitamins (like B5, B6, and folate).

- **Minerals**: They contain potassium, which helps maintain healthy blood pressure levels, magnesium, and copper, which support various body functions.

## 3. High in Fiber

- **Supports Digestive Health**: Avocados are a good source of dietary fiber, with around 10 grams of fiber per avocado. Fiber helps promote healthy digestion by adding bulk to stool, improving regularity, and preventing constipation.

- **Helps Control Blood Sugar**: The fiber in avocados also helps stabilize blood sugar levels by slowing the digestion and absorption of sugars, which can help prevent spikes in blood glucose after meals.

## 4. Supports Heart Health

- **Improves Cholesterol Levels**: Studies have shown that consuming avocados can help lower total cholesterol levels and LDL cholesterol, while increasing HDL (good) cholesterol, which is beneficial for overall heart health.

- **Rich in Potassium**: Avocados contain more potassium than bananas, a mineral that helps regulate blood pressure and supports healthy heart function.

## 5. Promotes Healthy Skin

- **Rich in Antioxidants**: Avocados contain antioxidants like vitamin E, vitamin C, and carotenoids, which help protect the skin from oxidative damage and support skin elasticity.

- **Hydrating**: The healthy fats in avocados help hydrate the skin, making it softer and more moisturized. Topically, avocado oil is often used in skincare products for its soothing and nourishing properties.

## 6. Supports Weight Management

- **Satiety**: Avocados are nutrient-dense and high in healthy fats and fiber, both of which help increase feelings of fullness and reduce overall calorie intake, making them beneficial for weight management.

- **Stable Blood Sugar**: Due to their low glycemic index and fiber content, avocados can help maintain stable blood sugar levels, which may reduce cravings and prevent overeating.

## 7. Rich in Antioxidants

- **Lutein and Zeaxanthin**: These antioxidants, found in avocados, are important for eye health. They help protect against oxidative stress and may reduce the risk of age-related macular degeneration and cataracts.

- **Protects Against Free Radical Damage**: The high levels of antioxidants in avocados help protect cells from free radical damage, reducing the risk of chronic diseases such as cancer and cardiovascular disease.

## 8. Improves Nutrient Absorption

- **Enhances Absorption of Fat-Soluble Nutrients**: The healthy fats in avocados help enhance the absorption of fat-soluble vitamins and nutrients, such as vitamins A, D, E, and K. Adding avocado to salads or vegetables can help your body absorb more of these nutrients.

## 9. Anti-Inflammatory Properties

- **Reduces Inflammation**: The monounsaturated fats, antioxidants, and phytochemicals in avocados help reduce inflammation in the body. Chronic inflammation is linked to conditions such as arthritis, heart disease, and diabetes, so reducing it can have significant health benefits.

## 10. Supports Brain Health

- **Rich in Healthy Fats**: Healthy fats in avocados support brain function by providing essential fatty acids that contribute to the structure and function of brain cells.

- **Folate**: Avocados are a good source of folate, which is important for brain development and function, and may help protect against cognitive decline and neurodegenerative diseases like Alzheimer's.

## 11. Supports Bone Health

- **Rich in Vitamin K**: Avocados are a good source of vitamin K, which plays an essential role in bone health by supporting calcium absorption and bone mineralization.

- **Other Nutrients**: Potassium, magnesium, and phosphorus content in avocados also contribute to maintaining healthy bones and joints.

## 12. Helps Detoxify the Body

- **Supports Liver Function**: Avocados have been shown to have liver-protective effects. They may help the liver detoxify and flush out harmful substances, supporting overall liver health.

- **Alkalizing**: The nutrients in avocados help balance the body's pH levels, making it less acidic, which supports overall detoxification processes.

## 13. Boosts Immune System

- **Vitamin C**: The vitamin C in avocados helps boost the immune system by supporting the production of white blood cells, which are essential for fighting infections.

- **Anti-inflammatory Properties**: By reducing inflammation, avocados support the immune system in fighting off infections and diseases more effectively.

## 14. May Reduce the Risk of Chronic Diseases

- **Cancer Prevention**: Some studies suggest that the antioxidants and anti-inflammatory properties in avocados may help reduce the risk of certain cancers by preventing oxidative damage and reducing inflammation in the body.

- **Diabetes Management**: The combination of fiber and healthy fats in avocados helps regulate blood sugar and insulin sensitivity, which can reduce the risk of type 2 diabetes or help manage the condition in those already diagnosed.

## Sprouted Tofu

I have been dissuaded from eating tofu because it is "bad" for me. The reason they say is due to it being estrogen-producing, or something like that. Guess what? I'm a woman, and estrogen has not bothered me a bit. This advice has come to me from meat-eaters usually. To them I say, "You eat dead animals, so please refrain from giving me advice." For men, if you don't want to take in extra estrogen, I overstand. For me, protein and calcium from tofu are ok for me! I've recently learned about soy's impact on the thyroid gland, and for that reason, I have a mind to start consuming soy in moderation.

Sprouted tofu has some unique benefits compared to regular tofu, thanks to the sprouting process the soybeans go through before being made into tofu. Here are the key perks:

1. **Easier to digest**: Sprouting helps break down some of the complex sugars and antinutrients (like **phytic acid**) in soybeans, which can make sprouted tofu gentler on the digestive system.

2. **Better nutrient absorption**: Because of the reduction in antinutrients, your body may absorb more minerals like calcium, iron, and zinc from sprouted tofu.

3. **Higher in protein (sometimes)**: Some brands of sprouted tofu contain slightly more protein per serving compared to regular tofu.

4. **Rich in enzymes**: The sprouting process activates beneficial enzymes that can support gut health and improve digestion.

5. **Retains all the tofu benefits**: Like regular tofu, it's still a great source of plant-based protein, calcium, and isoflavones (plant compounds with antioxidant properties).

Tofu, also known as bean curd, is a versatile and nutritious food made from soybeans. It is widely used in vegetarian and vegan diets as a plant-based protein source. Tofu is low in calories but packed with essential nutrients, offering a variety of health benefits. Here are some of the key benefits of tofu:

## 1. Excellent Source of Plant-Based Protein

- High-Quality Protein: Tofu is a great source of plant-based protein, which is essential for muscle growth, tissue repair, and overall body function. A 4-ounce serving of tofu provides around 10 grams of protein.

- Complete Protein: Unlike some plant-based proteins, tofu contains all nine essential amino acids, making it a complete protein source—ideal for vegetarians and vegans.

## 2. Rich in Nutrients

- Vitamins and Minerals: Tofu is rich in several important nutrients, including:

  o Iron: Essential for oxygen transport and preventing anemia.

  o Calcium: Vital for bone health and muscle function.

- o Magnesium: Supports nerve function, muscle health, and energy production.

- o Manganese: Important for bone health and metabolism.

## 3. Heart Health

- Cholesterol-Free: Tofu is a cholesterol-free food, which is beneficial for heart health. Replacing animal-based proteins with plant-based proteins like tofu may help lower cholesterol levels and reduce the risk of heart disease.

- Good Fats: Tofu contains healthy fats, including unsaturated fats, which can help improve blood lipid profiles and support heart health by reducing bad cholesterol (LDL) and increasing good cholesterol (HDL).

## 4. Supports Bone Health

- Rich in Calcium: Some varieties of tofu are fortified with calcium, which is important for maintaining strong bones and preventing osteoporosis.

- Magnesium and Phosphorus: Tofu also contains magnesium and phosphorus, both of which play a key role in bone formation and maintenance.

- Isoflavones: The phytoestrogens (plant estrogens) found in tofu, particularly isoflavones, may help improve bone density, especially in postmenopausal women, potentially reducing the risk of bone loss.

## 5. Supports Weight Management

- Low in Calories: Tofu is low in calories but high in protein, which can help you feel full and satisfied, preventing overeating, and promoting weight management.

- Rich in Fiber: Tofu contains some fiber, which aids digestion and helps with weight management by promoting satiety and reducing overall calorie intake.

## 6. Good for Digestive Health

- Gut Health: Tofu is made from soybeans, which contain beneficial compounds like phytochemicals and fiber that promote healthy digestion.

- Prebiotic Effect: The fiber in tofu acts as a prebiotic, promoting the growth of beneficial bacteria in the gut, which is crucial for a healthy microbiome and digestion.

## 7. Improves Skin Health

- Rich in Antioxidants: The isoflavones in tofu, specifically genistein and daidzein, have antioxidant properties that may help protect the skin from free radical damage and promote youthful, glowing skin.

- Collagen Production: Isoflavones in tofu can also stimulate collagen production, which is important for maintaining skin elasticity and reducing the appearance of wrinkles.

## 8. May Help Regulate Hormones

- Phytoestrogens: Tofu contains phytoestrogens, which are plant-based compounds that mimic the effects of estrogen in the body. These compounds may help regulate hormonal balance, particularly in women, by reducing symptoms related to menopause, such as hot flashes and mood swings.

- May Reduce Menopausal Symptoms: Studies have shown that consuming soy products like tofu can help reduce menopausal symptoms by balancing hormone levels.

I have been eating tofu for decades, and now that I am past the age of 50, fortunately, there have been no menopause symptoms in sight!

## 9. Supports Healthy Blood Sugar Levels

- Low Glycemic Index: Tofu has a low glycemic index, meaning it has a minimal impact on blood sugar levels. This makes it an excellent choice for people with diabetes or those looking to maintain stable blood sugar.

- Helps Improve Insulin Sensitivity: Some studies suggest that soy-based products like tofu may help improve insulin sensitivity, which can lower the risk of type 2 diabetes.

## 10. Cancer Prevention

- Isoflavones and Antioxidants: The isoflavones in tofu have been studied for their potential cancer-fighting properties. These compounds may help inhibit the growth of certain types of cancer cells, particularly breast and prostate cancer.

- Lignans: Tofu also contains lignans, which are antioxidant-rich compounds that may help protect against cancer by reducing oxidative stress and inflammation.

## 11. Anti-Inflammatory Properties

- Reduces Inflammation: The compounds found in tofu, including isoflavones and antioxidants, may help reduce inflammation in the body. Chronic inflammation is linked to many conditions, including heart disease, arthritis, and cancer, so consuming anti-inflammatory foods like tofu may lower the risk of these diseases.

## 12. Good for Kidney Health

- Kidney Disease Management: Tofu, being a plant-based protein, may be a better option than animal-based proteins for individuals with kidney disease, as it places less strain on the kidneys and can help manage symptoms of kidney dysfunction.

## Toasted Sesame Oil

Toasted sesame oil is a flavorful oil made from roasted sesame seeds. It's commonly used in Asian cuisine for its distinct, nutty taste and rich aroma. In addition to enhancing the flavor of various dishes, toasted sesame oil offers a variety of health benefits. Here are some of the key benefits of toasted sesame oil:

## 1. Rich in Healthy Fats

- **Monounsaturated and Polyunsaturated Fats**: Toasted sesame oil is a good source of healthy fats, particularly monounsaturated fats (like oleic acid) and polyunsaturated fats (like linoleic acid). These fats help reduce bad cholesterol (LDL) levels and support heart health.

- **Supports Heart Health**: The healthy fats in toasted sesame oil help improve blood lipid profiles and reduce the risk of cardiovascular diseases when consumed in moderation.

## 2. High in Antioxidants

- **Sesamol and Sesamin**: Toasted sesame oil is rich in powerful antioxidants like sesamol and sesamin, which help protect the body from oxidative stress by neutralizing free radicals. These antioxidants contribute to reducing the risk of chronic diseases such as heart disease, cancer, and diabetes.

- **Protects Cells**: The antioxidants in sesame oil help prevent cellular damage and inflammation, promoting overall cellular health and longevity.

## 3. Anti-Inflammatory Properties

- **Reduces Inflammation**: The compounds found in toasted sesame oil, including sesamin, have natural anti-inflammatory effects. This can help reduce inflammation in the body, which is beneficial for conditions like arthritis, joint pain, and other inflammatory diseases.

## 4. Supports Skin Health

- **Rich in Vitamin E**: Toasted sesame oil contains vitamin E, an essential nutrient that supports skin health by protecting the skin from oxidative damage caused by UV rays and environmental stressors.

- **Moisturizes and Nourishes**: The oil's fatty acids and antioxidants help hydrate and nourish the skin, making it a popular ingredient in skin-care products. It also has the potential to reduce the appearance of wrinkles and fine lines.

- **Anti-Aging Effects**: The high levels of antioxidants, particularly sesamol, may help slow down the aging process by protecting skin cells from damage and promoting collagen production.

## 5. Promotes Healthy Hair

- **Moisturizes Hair**: The fatty acids in toasted sesame oil help to nourish and moisturize dry hair, making it softer and shinier.

- **Scalp Health**: It can help improve scalp health by soothing dry, flaky skin and may also help reduce dandruff.

- **Strengthens Hair**: Regular use of sesame oil on hair may help strengthen hair follicles and reduce hair breakage, promoting healthy, thicker hair growth.

## 6. Supports Bone Health

- **Rich in Calcium**: Sesame oil contains calcium, an essential mineral for strong and healthy bones. Adequate calcium intake helps prevent bone-related disorders like osteoporosis.

- **Magnesium**: Sesame oil also contains magnesium, which plays a vital role in bone health and helps regulate the metabolism of calcium.

## 7. May Lower Blood Pressure

- **Lowers Blood Pressure**: Some studies suggest that sesame oil may help lower high blood pressure due to its ability to relax blood vessels and improve circulation. The oil's polyunsaturated fats, especially omega-6 fatty acids, may be responsible for this effect.

## 8. Good for Digestion

- **Promotes Digestive Health**: The oil has mild laxative effects, which can promote better digestion and relieve constipation.

- **Soothes the Digestive Tract**: Sesame oil has been traditionally used to soothe inflammation in the digestive tract and reduce symptoms of conditions like acid reflux and gastritis.

## 9. Supports Immune Health

- **Rich in Zinc**: Zinc is essential for a healthy immune system, and sesame oil provides a source of this vital mineral.

- **Anti-viral and Anti-bacterial Properties**: Some studies suggest that sesame oil may have mild antimicrobial properties, helping to support the body's defenses against infections.

## 10. Helps Manage Blood Sugar Levels

- **Blood Sugar Regulation**: Some research indicates that sesame oil may help lower blood sugar levels, which is beneficial for people with diabetes or those at risk of developing the condition. Its ability to improve insulin sensitivity can support better blood sugar management.

## 11. May Improve Heart Health

- **Lowers Cholesterol**: The compounds found in sesame oil, including sesamin and sesamol, may help reduce cholesterol levels in the blood, thus supporting heart health by lowering the risk of heart disease.

- **Improves Circulation**: The oil's fatty acids help improve circulation and reduce the risk of blood clot formation.

## 12. Helps with Stress and Anxiety

- **Calming Effects**: Some studies suggest that sesame oil may have a calming effect on the nervous system, potentially helping reduce anxiety and stress. It has been used in traditional medicine for its potential to soothe the mind and body.

## Fresh Squeezed Lemon Juice

is a popular and refreshing beverage known for its tangy flavor, but it also offers a wide range of health benefits. Packed with essential vitamins, minerals, and antioxidants, lemon juice can be a great addition to a healthy lifestyle. Here are some of the key benefits of lemon juice:

## 1. Rich in Vitamin C

- Boosts Immunity: Lemon juice is an excellent source of vitamin C, a powerful antioxidant that helps strengthen the immune system. Vitamin C can help the body fight off infections and illnesses, such as the common cold.

- Supports Collagen Production: Vitamin C plays a crucial role in collagen synthesis, which is essential for healthy skin, blood vessels, and connective tissues.

## 2. Supports Digestive Health

- Aids Digestion: Lemon juice can help promote better digestion by stimulating the production of digestive enzymes. It can also help relieve symptoms like indigestion and bloating.

- Alkalizing Effect: Although lemon juice is acidic, it has an alkalizing effect on the body once metabolized. This can help balance pH levels in the stomach and improve overall digestion.

- Relieves Constipation: Drinking lemon juice with warm water in the morning can act as a mild natural laxative, promoting regular bowel movements and preventing constipation.

## 3. Hydration and Detoxification

- Hydrates the Body: Lemon juice, when added to water, enhances hydration due to its refreshing taste, making it easier to drink more water throughout the day.

- Detoxifies the Body: Lemon juice can promote detoxification by stimulating the liver to produce bile, which is essential for digestion and the removal of toxins from the body. It also acts as a natural diuretic, helping to flush out excess fluids.

## 4. Rich in Antioxidants

- Fights Free Radicals: Lemon juice contains antioxidants like flavonoids and vitamin C that help combat oxidative stress and reduce the damage caused by free radicals. This can help lower the risk of chronic diseases like heart disease and cancer.

- Protects Skin Health: The antioxidants in lemon juice can help protect the skin from UV damage and premature aging, contributing to a healthy and youthful appearance.

## 5. Supports Weight Loss

- Boosts Metabolism: Drinking lemon juice can increase metabolism, helping the body burn fat more efficiently. The pectin fiber found in lemons may also help reduce hunger cravings and promote feelings of fullness.

- Detox and Cleansing: Lemon juice's detoxifying properties can help cleanse the body, promoting better digestion and reducing bloating, which may support weight management.

## 6. Improves Skin Health

- Fights Acne: The antibacterial properties of lemon juice can help fight acne and reduce inflammation. When applied topically (with caution), lemon juice can help cleanse the skin and reduce the occurrence of blemishes and breakouts.

- Brightens Skin: Vitamin C in lemon juice helps reduce skin pigmentation and discoloration, promoting a more even skin tone. It also helps in collagen formation, which can improve skin elasticity and reduce the appearance of fine lines and wrinkles.

- Reduces Dark Spots: Regular use of lemon juice may help fade dark spots, age spots, and freckles due to its ability to lighten the skin.

## 7. Improves Oral Health

- Freshens Breath: Lemon juice helps freshen your breath by neutralizing odors in the mouth. The acidity in lemon juice also stimulates saliva production, which helps to cleanse the mouth and maintain oral hygiene.

- Fights Plaque and Tartar: Lemon juice has natural antibacterial properties that can help reduce plaque buildup and fight harmful bacteria in the mouth. However, it's important to use lemon juice in moderation to prevent enamel erosion due to its acidity.

## 8. Boosts Heart Health

- Promotes Healthy Blood Pressure: Lemon juice contains potassium, which can help regulate blood pressure by balancing sodium levels in the body.

- Supports Cholesterol Levels: Some studies suggest that lemon juice can help lower "bad" LDL cholesterol levels while increasing "good" HDL cholesterol, promoting overall heart health.

- Antioxidant Protection: The antioxidants in lemon juice may also help protect the heart by reducing inflammation and oxidative damage that could contribute to cardiovascular diseases.

## 9. Balances pH Levels

- Alkalizes the Body: While lemon juice is acidic in nature, it has an alkalizing effect on the body once metabolized. Maintaining a balanced pH is important for overall health, as an overly acidic environment in the body can lead to inflammation and other health issues.

### 10. Helps with Respiratory Health

- Soothes Sore Throat: Lemon juice has antibacterial properties that can help soothe a sore throat and reduce irritation. It can be mixed with honey and warm water for a calming remedy.

- Relieves Congestion: The vitamin C in lemon juice can help boost the immune system, which can support the body in fighting off respiratory infections like colds or flu. It may also help relieve congestion.

### 11. Improves Mood and Energy

- Boosts Mood: The refreshing scent and acidity of lemon juice can have mood-boosting effects. The scent of lemon has been shown to have a calming effect, reduce stress, and increase feelings of happiness and alertness.

- Increases Energy: The high vitamin C content in lemon juice can reduce fatigue and improve energy levels. It helps the body absorb iron from plant-based foods, which is important for maintaining energy and preventing anemia.

## Food Don'ts

### Sodium control

Salty food is a big-time norm in just about all foods we purchase from the store or get at fast food restaurants. Just read the back of any canned food. The sodium levels are usually through the roof! The salt is how they are able to store the food for so long. The salt serves as a preservative. I never paid too much attention to the sodium content of food. I didn't believe the sodium fact really pertained to me. Now that I have high blood pressure concerns, I am learning to monitor the sodium content of foods like a hawk! Not only are there massive amounts of sodium in canned foods, but I also found that I had to really read the labels of my spices as well. Oh, how I had to get rid of spices I loved. My blood pressure was trending high every night, yet when I ceased using spices high in sodium, my blood pressure went down. Take heed to the salt content in your food. It's in more than I bet you imagine.

## MSG (Monosodium Glutamate)

There is MSG in tons of food. It is a flavor enhancer. When I would go to the Chinese restaurant, I knew enough to ask them not to add MSG to my food. Recently, I had to get rid of my most desired spice because it contained MSG. That good taste is not worth the insidious effects MSG can have on our bodies. Here is some important information to know about MSG:

Monosodium glutamate (MSG) is a flavor enhancer commonly added to foods like soups, canned vegetables, snacks, and restaurant dishes. It's known for giving food that tastes **savory**.

Some people report mild, short-term symptoms after consuming large amounts of MSG, often called "MSG Symptom Complex" or "Chinese Restaurant Syndrome."

- Headache
- Flushing
- Sweating
- Facial pressure or tightness
- Numbness or tingling
- Chest pain
- Nausea
- Weakness

These symptoms usually go away on their own and are not considered dangerous.

- There's been speculation that MSG could affect the brain or contribute to conditions like migraines, but scientific evidence doesn't support strong links in healthy individuals.

- Some animal studies suggested high doses might affect brain cells, but those doses were much higher than what people consume in food.

- People with asthma, migraines, or histamine intolerance might be more likely to react to MSG.

- Children might also be more sensitive in some cases, though again, evidence is mixed.

MSG can appear under different names on labels:

- Hydrolyzed protein
- Yeast extract
- Glutamic acid
- "Natural flavoring"

# A GOOD NIGHT'S REST & NEGATIVE IONS

I don't think folks value a good night's rest until they don't get one. Our body heals when we sleep. If my pressure was high, I actually couldn't sleep. It was the worst. I would switch from lying on my couch with "Little House on the Prairie" in the background to my bed with the window cracked and a heating pad under my covers to keep my feet warm. If my pressure was high going to sleep, it was usually accompanied by high sugar. Once I got both of these things under control through insulin and medicine, I could finally fall asleep.

One thing that helped me fall asleep were the waves of Lake Michigan outside my window. Now you might think that the sound of crashing waves made me sleepy, but that wasn't it. Moving water gives off negative ions. What are negative ions?

Negative ions, often found in nature (especially around waterfalls, mountains, oceans, and forests), are molecules that have gained an extra electron, giving them a negative charge. Research shows that negative ions can have various health and wellness benefits. Here are some of the commonly reported benefits:

## 1. Improved Mood

- Negative ions may increase levels of serotonin, the "feel-good" neurotransmitter.
- This can help reduce feelings of depression, anxiety, and stress.

## 2. Better Sleep

- Some studies suggest that negative ions can help regulate melatonin levels, which may improve sleep quality.

### 3. Enhanced Mental Clarity & Focus

- People often report feeling more alert and clear-headed after exposure to negative ions.
- This might be due to increased oxygen flow to the brain.

### 4. Air Purification

- Negative ions bind to airborne particles like dust, pollen, smoke, and dander, causing them to fall to the ground.
- This can reduce allergens and pollutants in the air, potentially benefiting people with asthma or allergies.

### 5. Increased Energy

- Especially when experienced in natural environments, negative ions can create a sense of refreshment or a "natural high."

### 6. Reduced Inflammation & Oxidative Stress (Potential)

- There's emerging research suggesting they might have antioxidant-like properties, helping to combat oxidative stress, though more evidence is needed.

Sleeping with my window cracked to get the negative ions coming from Lake Michigan works like a charm. I experience deep sleep every time I have the negative ion opportunity. There are apparently negative ion generators you can investigate, but I don't know their effectiveness. I am extremely grateful for access to negative ions as part of my healing regimen.

# Summary

I'm a teacher at heart, and I share what I learn with those around me. This healing journey has been moments of ebbs, flows, and learning that I felt like I had to share it. I have faith that my viewpoints are helpful, and my research tells you things you may not have known. Use the data in this book if it matches what you want for yourself and your loved ones. When talking about my health challenges, one of my friends said to me, "You just don't know what you don't know." This book was written to help increase knowingness for all who read it. It is replete with my truths and may complement your own health journey.

The major key is to be responsible for the quality of your life...when you're ready. I suggest not waiting for adversity and times of challenge to make you ready. CHOOSE health. CHOOSE happiness. CHOOSE courage. CHOOSE wisdom. CHOOSE to listen. CHOOSE to act. CHOOSE discipline. CHOOSE good decisions. CHOOSE God. CHOOSE yourself.

I Had to CHOOSE to Feel Better

# Glossary

**A1C (n.) -** (also written as HbA1c) is a blood test that measures your average blood sugar (glucose) levels over the past 2 to 3 months. It's commonly used to diagnose and monitor diabetes. Below 5.7% - Normal, 5.7% – 6.4% - Prediabetes, 6.6% or higher – Diabetes (type 1or type 2)

**abdomen** (n.) -The part of the body of a vertebrate between the thorax (chest) and the pelvis, containing the digestive organs.

**absorption** (n.) - The process of taking in a substance (such as a liquid or gas) by chemical or physical action.

**accumulate** (v.) - To gather or collect something over time.

**acetic acid** (n.) - A colorless organic acid with a sharp, sour taste and strong smell, used in the production of vinegar and as a chemical reagent.

**Acid Reflux** (n.) - A medical condition in which stomach acid flows back into the esophagus, causing symptoms like heartburn or indigestion.

**acne** (n.) - A skin condition that occurs when hair follicles become clogged with oil and dead skin cells, often resulting in pimples, blackheads, or cysts.

**ACV (Apple Cider Vinegar)** (n.) - a type of vinegar made from fermented apple juice, commonly used in cooking, cleaning, and sometimes as a health remedy.

**adaptogenic** (adj.) Describing a substance (usually an herb or plant) believed to help the body resist stressors of all kinds — physical, chemical, or biological.

**adenosine** (n.) - A naturally occurring chemical in the body that plays a role in energy transfer (as part of ATP) and signaling in the brain and heart.

**adequate** (adj.) - sufficient for a specific requirement or purpose.

**ADHD (Attention-Deficit/Hyperactivity Disorder) (n.)** - A neurodevelopmental disorder characterized by symptoms of inattention, hyperactivity, and impulsivity **that interfere with functioning or development.**

**adoration** (n.) - deep love, respect, or worship for someone or something.

**adrenal glands** (n.) - The adrenal glands are two small, triangular-shaped glands located on top of each kidney. They are part of your endocrine system and produce hormones that help regulate key body functions like stress response, metabolism, blood pressure, and salt balance.

**adrenal medulla (n.)** - is the inner part of the adrenal glands, which are small glands located on top of your kidneys. The adrenal glands have two main parts: the outer part, called the adrenal cortex, and the inner part, the adrenal medulla. The adrenal medulla is primarily responsible for the production and release of important hormones known as catecholamines, including:

- **Adrenaline (epinephrine)**
- **Norepinephrine (noradrenaline)**

These hormones are involved in the body's fight-or-flight response, helping you react to stress or danger.

**Adrenaline (n.)**, also known as epinephrine, is a hormone and neurotransmitter produced by the adrenal glands, specifically in the adrenal medulla (the inner part of the adrenal glands). It plays a crucial role in the body's fight-or-flight response, which helps you respond to stress or danger.

**adversity** (n.) - Difficulties or misfortune; a condition marked by hardship or suffering.

**advocate (n.)** – a person who speaks or writes in support or defense of a person or cause

**aesthetic** (adj.) - concerned with beauty or the appreciation of beauty.

**Aldosterone (n.)** - is a hormone produced by the adrenal glands (specifically the adrenal cortex) that plays a crucial role in regulating blood pressure, blood volume, and electrolyte balance, especially the levels of sodium ($Na^+$) and potassium ($K^+$) in the body.

**alkaline** (adj.) - having a pH greater than 7; the opposite of acidic

**alkalizing** (adj.) - having the property or effect of making something more alkaline

**Alkamides** (n.) - are a class of naturally occurring bioactive compounds, primarily found in plants such as Echinacea. They are known for their lipid-like structure and are often studied for their effects on the immune system and nervous system.

**alleviate** (v.) - to reduce, ease, or relieve pain, suffering, or a burden.

**allicin** – (n.) - A sulfur-containing compound produced when garlic is crushed or chopped, known for its distinctive smell, and believed health benefits

**alpha-linolenic acid (ALA)** (n.) - An essential omega-3 fatty acid found in plant sources like flaxseed, chia seeds, walnuts, and canola oil.

**Alzheimer's Disease (n.)** - A progressive neurodegenerative disease that causes memory loss, cognitive decline, and behavioral changes, most commonly affecting older adults.

**amino acids** (n.) - Organic compounds that serve as the building blocks of proteins

**Androgens** (n.) - are a group of hormones that play a key role in the development of male characteristics and the regulation of reproductive activity. While they are often referred to as "male hormones," androgens are present in both males and females, though at different levels.

**anemia** (n.) - A medical condition in which the body lacks enough healthy red blood cells or hemoglobin, resulting in reduced oxygen transport to the body's tissues

**Anthocyanins** (n.) - Natural pigments found in plants that give red, purple, and blue colors to fruits, vegetables, and flowers.

**Antibacterial** (adj.) - Preventing the growth of or destroying bacteria.

**Antifungal** (adj.) - Preventing the growth of or destroying fungi.

**antiviral** (adj.) - Acting to prevent or treat viral infections

**anti-inflammatories** (n.) - Drugs or substances that reduce inflammation or swelling in the body.

**antioxidants** (n.) - Substances that inhibit oxidation and neutralize free radicals, which can damage cells.

**anxiety** (n.) - A feeling of worry, nervousness, or unease, typically about something with an uncertain outcome.

**anxious** (adj.) - Experiencing worry, unease, or nervousness, typically about an event that's likely to happen or something with an uncertain outcome.

**arrhythmias** (n.) - irregular heartbeats

**arterial** (adj.) - Relating to an artery or arteries.

**arteries** (n.) - Blood vessels that carry oxygen-rich blood away from the heart to the body

**arthritic** (adj.) – related to, having, or experiencing chronic inflammation of a joint, often accompanied by pain and structural changes and infection or injury or injury.

arthritis (n.) - A medical condition involving inflammation of one or more joints, causing pain, swelling, and stiffness.

**artichoke** (n.) - A vegetable with a large, edible flower bud, typically cooked and eaten before the flower blooms.

**articulate** (v.) - to give clarity or the recognizing or noting of differences

**arugula** (n.) - A leafy green vegetable with a peppery, slightly bitter flavor, often used in salads.

**Ashwagandha** (n.) - An herb used in traditional Ayurvedic medicine, known for its adaptogenic properties (helps the body manage stress).

**assessment** (n.) - evaluation

**assignment** (n.) - a position of responsibility, post of duty, or the like, to which one is appointed

**associated** (adj.) - Connected or related to something else.

**asthma** (n.) - A chronic respiratory condition marked by inflammation and narrowing of the airways, causing wheezing, shortness of breath, coughing, and chest tightness.

**atomic** (adj.) - Relating to atoms, the basic units of matter.

**ATP** (adenosine triphosphate) (n.) - the main energy carrier in cells

**atrocious (adj.) -** shockingly bad or tasteless; dreadful

**authority (n.) -** an expert on a subject

**autoimmune** (adj.) - Relating to a condition in which the immune system mistakenly attacks the body's own tissues.

**autonomic nervous system (n.) - (ANS)** is the part of your nervous system that automatically controls involuntary body functions, meaning it operates without you having to think about it. It regulates things like heart rate, breathing, digestion, blood pressure, pupil size, and body temperature — all critical for survival and homeostasis.

**aware** (adj.) – having knowledge; mindful

**bacteria** (n.) - Microscopic single-celled organisms that exist in various environments, some of which cause disease, while others are beneficial.

**bad cholesterol (LDL)** (n.) - carries cholesterol from the liver to cells. If too much is delivered, it can build up in the walls of arteries.

**bananas** (adj.) - The slang word "bananas" means crazy, wild, or extremely irrational — either in a funny or chaotic way, depending on the context.

**Berberine** (n.) - A natural compound found in several plants (e.g., goldenseal, barberry), known for its antimicrobial and metabolic health properties. Helps with sugar control

**beta-carotene** (n.) - A red-orange pigment found in plants and fruits (especially carrots), which the body can convert into vitamin A.

**beta-glucans** (n.) - Soluble fibers found in oats, barley, mushrooms, and yeast, known to support immune function and lower cholesterol.

**bile** (n.) - A digestive fluid produced by the liver and stored in the gallbladder, which helps break down fats in the small intestine.

**Bladderwrack** (n.) - A type of brown seaweed (Fucus vesiculosus) rich in iodine, used traditionally for thyroid support and weight loss.

**bioenergetics** (adj.) - the study of energy transformation in living systems.

**Blood Pressure** (n.) - is the force of blood pushing against the walls of your arteries as your heart pumps it through your body. It's a key measure of your heart and blood vessel health.

**blue light damage** (n.) - Potential harm to the eyes and skin caused by prolonged exposure to high-energy visible (HEV) blue light, commonly emitted from screens (phones, tablets, computers) and LED lighting.

**Body Comm (Communication) (n.) -** Place your hands in different positions on the body, giving a command and acknowledging the person each time after he has responded. The purpose of the process is to enable the being to reestablish communication with his body.

**bolster** (v.) - To support, strengthen, or reinforce.

**bone mineral density** (n.) - A measurement of the amount of minerals (primarily calcium and phosphorus) contained in a specific volume of bone.

**Burdock Root** (n.) - The root of the burdock plant (*Arctium lappa*), traditionally used in herbal medicine for detoxification, skin health, and digestion.

**caffeine** (n.) - is a natural stimulant found in coffee, tea, cacao (chocolate), energy drinks, and some medications. It primarily affects the central nervous system, helping you feel more alert, awake, and energetic by blocking a chemical in the brain called adenosine, which normally makes you feel tired.

**Calcium** (n.) – A chemical element (symbol: Ca) essential for healthy bones, teeth, muscle function, nerve signaling, and blood clotting.

**calorie** (n.) - A unit of energy; in nutrition, it refers to the amount of energy a food provides.

**cancer cells** (n.) - Abnormal cells that divide uncontrollably and can invade nearby tissues or spread throughout the body.

**capacity** (n.) - The role or function in which someone acts

**capers** (n.) - The pickled flower buds of the caper bush, used as a tangy seasoning in cooking.

**carbohydrate** (n.) - A macronutrient composed of carbon, hydrogen, and oxygen that provides energy for the body, especially in the form of sugars, starches, and fibers.

**carbon** – **(n.)** a widely distributed element that forms organic compounds in combination with hydrogen, oxygen, etc., and that occurs in a pure state as diamond and graphite, and in an impure state as charcoal.

**carcinogens** (n.) - Substances or agents capable of causing cancer in living tissue.

**cardiovascular** (adj.) - Relating to the heart and blood vessels.

**carotenoids** (n.) - Pigments found in plants and some animal tissues that have antioxidant properties and often provide red, yellow, or orange color (e.g., in carrots, tomatoes).

**casein** (n.) - The main protein found in milk and dairy products, known for slow digestion.

**cataracts** (n.) - A medical condition in which the lens of the eye becomes cloudy, leading to impaired vision.

**catechins** (n.) - A type of natural antioxidant (flavonoid) found in tea, cocoa, berries, and apples, known for its health-promoting properties.

**catecholamines** (n.) - are a group of hormones and neurotransmitters that are produced by the adrenal glands (specifically the adrenal medulla) and nerve cells. Catecholamines play a critical role in the body's stress response and regulate functions such as heart rate, blood pressure, and energy production.

**cause** (v.) – to bring about

**celiac disease** (n.) - An autoimmune disorder in which the ingestion of gluten (a protein in wheat, barley, and rye) damages the small intestine lining.

**ceylon cinnamon** (n.) - A type of cinnamon (from the *Cinnamomum verum* tree), often called "true cinnamon," known for its mild flavor and lower coumarin content. It's known to assist with blood sugar management

**chia seeds** (n.) - Tiny edible seeds from the *Salvia hispanica* plant, rich in omega-3 fatty acids, fiber, protein, and antioxidants.

**cholesterol** (n.) - A waxy, fat-like substance found in all the cells of the body, essential for hormone production, vitamin D synthesis, and cell membrane structure.

**chlorophyll** (n.) - The green pigment in plants that absorbs sunlight for photosynthesis.

**choline** (n.) - An essential nutrient that supports brain development, liver function, muscle movement, and metabolism.

**chromium** (n.) - A trace mineral important for regulating blood sugar by enhancing the action of insulin.

**chronic** (adj.) - Having long had a disease, habit, weakness, or the like.

**circadian** (adj.) - Relating to biological processes that follow a 24-hour cycle, such as the sleep-wake rhythm.

**circulation** (n.) - The continuous movement of blood through the heart and blood vessels, delivering oxygen and nutrients throughout the body.

**circulatory** (adj.) - Relating to the circulation of blood or lymph through the body.

**circumstance** (n.) - an incident or occurrence.

**claustrophobic** (adj.) - Having an irrational fear of confined or enclosed spaces.

**cognitive** (adj.) - Relating to the mental processes of perception, memory, judgment, reasoning, and learning.

**collagen** (n.) - A structural protein found in skin, bones, tendons, and connective tissues that provides strength and elasticity.

**colon** (n.) - The final part of the digestive system (large intestine), where water is absorbed and waste is stored before elimination.

**commercial** (adj.) - Related to business, trade, or commerce.

**compounds** (n.) - Substances made from two or more different elements chemically bonded together.

**comprehensive** (adj.) - covering or involving much; inclusive.

**condiment** (n.) - A seasoning or sauce served at the table or added during food preparation.

**congestive heart failure (CHF)** (n.) - A chronic condition where the heart is unable to pump blood effectively, leading to fluid buildup in the lungs, legs, and other tissues.

**constipation** (n.) - a condition of the bowels in which the feces are dry and hardened and evacuation is difficult and infrequent.

**consumption** (n.) - The act of using, eating, or drinking something.

**conventional** (adj.) - Based on or in accordance with what is generally done or believed; traditional or standard.

**copper** (n.) - An essential trace mineral important for red blood cell production and immune function.

**coronary** (adj.) - Relating to the arteries that supply blood to the heart muscle.

**correlation** (n.) - mutual relation of two or more things, parts, etc.

**cortisol** (n.) - is a hormone made by your adrenal glands, located on top of your kidneys. It's often called the "stress hormone" because it's released in response to stress, but it also plays important roles in metabolism, immune function, blood pressure, and blood sugar regulation.

**creditable** (adj.) - bringing or deserving credit, honor.

**CRP(C-reactive protein)** (n.) - A protein made by the liver and released into the blood in response to inflammation.

**crucial** (adj.) - Extremely important or essential.

**cuisine** (n.) - The food of a particular culture or place.

**cytokines** (n.) - Small proteins released by cells, especially immune cells, that affect the behavior of other cells.

**daidzein** (n.) - A type of isoflavone (plant compound) found in soy and other legumes, with estrogen-like and antioxidant effects.

**dander** (n.) - Tiny flakes of skin shed by animals with fur or feathers, often causing allergic reactions.

**deficiency** (n.) – the state of lacking some element or characteristic; incompleteness.

**defy** (v.) - To resist or refuse to obey a rule, law, or authority.

**dehydration** (n.) - A condition that occurs when the body loses more fluids than it takes in, leading to a lack of water for normal functions.

**deja'vu** (n.) – The sense of feeling of having previously experienced something that really has been encountered before.

**Dementia** (n.) - A progressive neurological disorder affecting memory, thinking, and behavior.

**denial** (n.) - disbelief in the existence or reality of a thing.

**depression** (n.) - A mental health disorder marked by persistent sadness, loss of interest or pleasure, and other emotional and physical problems.

**detoxification** (n.) - The process of removing toxic substances or drugs from the body.

**detrimental** (adj.) - Having a negative effect on something.

**Diabetes (Type 1)** (n.) - A chronic condition in which the pancreas produces little or no insulin, usually diagnosed in childhood or adolescence.

**Diabetes (Type 2)** (n.) - A chronic condition affecting the way the body processes blood sugar (glucose), often linked to insulin resistance.

**diagnose** (v.) – to classify or determine based on scientific examination.

**digestion** (n.) - The process by which food is broken down in the body into nutrients the body can absorb and use.

**digestive system** (n.) - The system of organs responsible for breaking down food, absorbing nutrients, and eliminating waste.

**dilate** (v.) - To make wider or larger; to expand.

**discipline** (n.) - behavior in accord with rules of conduct; behavior and order maintained by training and control.

**disclaimer** (n.) – a statement or document that denies responsibility.

**discretion** (n.) - the power or right to decide or act according to one's own judgment, freedom of judgment or choice.

**diuretic** (n.) - A substance that increases urine production and helps remove excess water and salt from the body.

**diverticulosis** (n.) - A condition where small bulging pouches (diverticula) form in the lining of the digestive tract, especially the colon.

**dopamine** (n.) - is a neurotransmitter — a chemical messenger in the brain — that plays a major role in movement, motivation, mood, and reward.

**dousing** (n.) - The act of pouring liquid over something or someone.

**download** (n.) - data that has been transferred from a Higher spiritual source to a human source

**DNA (n.) - DNA** stands for deoxyribonucleic acid. It is the molecule that carries the genetic instructions used in the growth, development, functioning, and reproduction of all known living organisms and many viruses.

**DNA Synthesis** (n.) - The natural or artificial process of creating deoxyribonucleic acid (DNA) molecules.

**Dysbiosis** (n.) - An imbalance or unhealthy change in the gut microbiome, often linked to digestive or immune problems.

**echinacea** (n.) - is a genus of flowering plants in the daisy family (Asteraceae), native to North America. It is best known for its use in herbal medicine, especially for immune support and helping prevent or shorten the duration of colds and respiratory infections.

**echinacosides** (n.) - are a group of natural phenolic compounds (specifically, caffeic acid glycosides) primarily found in certain species of the Echinacea plant, especially Echinacea angustifolia and Echinacea pallida. They are considered one of the key bioactive components in echinacea-based herbal remedies.

**eczema** (n.) - A chronic skin condition that causes red, itchy, inflamed, or cracked skin.

**efficiently** (adv.) - In a way that achieves maximum productivity with minimum wasted effort or expense.

**elasticity** (n.) - The ability of an object or material to return to its original shape after being stretched or compressed.

**electrolyte** (n.) is a charged mineral (or ion) that dissolves in body fluids and helps regulate many essential bodily functions, including hydration, nerve signals, muscle function, and pH balance.

**electron** (n.) - A subatomic particle with a negative electric charge, found in all atoms and acting as the primary carrier of electricity in solids.

**ellagic acid** (n.) - A natural antioxidant compound found in fruits and vegetables like pomegranates, berries, and nuts.

**elongate** (v.) - To make something longer or stretch it out.

**endocrine system (n.)** - The endocrine system is a network of glands and organs that produce and release hormones — chemical messengers that help regulate many important body functions like growth, metabolism, mood, reproduction, and stress response.

**Energy Enhancement Center** (n.) – refers to wellness centers that utilize the Energy Enhancement System (EESystem), a technology designed to promote natural healing and wellness through advanced bioenergetic fields. These centers are equipped with specialized equipment that emits scalar waves and other frequencies to support the body's innate healing processes. (totallyuhealin.com – (331)-444-2709)

**entails** (v.) - To involve something as a necessary or inevitable part or consequence.

**entirety** (n.) - The whole of something; the complete thing.

**enzyme** (n.) – A biological molecule (typically a protein) that speeds up chemical reactions in living organisms.

**epilepsy** (n.) – a disorder of the nervous system, characterized either by mild episodic loss of attention or sleepiness or by severe convulsions with loss of consciousness.

**Epithelial lining** (n.) - refers to a layer of epithelial cells that forms a protective or functional surface on the inside or outside of body structures such as organs, blood vessels, and cavities.

**Functions of Epithelial Cells:**

| Function | Example Location | Description |
|----------|------------------|-------------|
| **Protection** | Skin, lining of mouth | Shields tissues from injury and pathogens |
| **Absorption** | Small intestine | Absorbs nutrients |
| **Secretion** | Glands (salivary, sweat) | Releases substances like enzymes, hormones, sweat |
| **Filtration** | Kidneys | Filters blood and forms urine |
| **Sensation** | Skin, nasal passages | Contains nerve endings for touch and smell |

**erosion** (n.) - The gradual destruction or wearing away of something by natural forces such as wind, water, or ice.

**eruption (n.) -** the breaking out of a rash or the like

**esophageal** (adj.) - Relating to the esophagus (the tube that carries food from the mouth to the stomach).

**esophagus** (n.) - The muscular tube in the body through which food passes from the throat to the stomach.

**essential** (adj.) - Absolutely necessary or extremely important.

**essential fatty acids** (n.) - Fatty acids that the body cannot produce on its own and must be obtained through the diet (e.g., omega-3 and omega-6).

**estrogen** (n.) - A group of hormones that play a key role in the development and regulation of the female reproductive system and secondary sex characteristics.

**evident** (adj.) - Clearly seen or understood; obvious.

**fasting blood sugar levels** (n.) - The concentration of glucose in the blood after a person has not eaten (fasted) for at least 8 hours.

**fat-soluble** (adj.) - Able to dissolve in or be absorbed with fats or oils.

**fatigue** (n.) - Extreme tiredness resulting from mental or physical exertion or illness.

**fatty acid** (n.) - A type of organic acid found in fats and oils, often used by the body for energy or to build cell membranes.

**fennel** (n.) - The bulb, seeds, or leaves of the fennel plant, used for culinary and medicinal purposes.

**fermented** (adj.) - Having undergone fermentation — a process in which sugars are converted to acids, gases, or alcohol by bacteria or yeast.

**fervor** (n.) - Intense and passionate feeling.

**fester** (v.) - To become worse or more intense over time, especially regarding emotions or problems.

**fetal neural tube** (n.) - A structure in the developing fetus that eventually forms the brain and spinal cord.

**fiber** (n.) - A type of carbohydrate found in plant foods that the body cannot digest, important for digestive health.

**fight-or-flight response (n.) -** is the body's natural reaction to stress, danger, or threatening situations. It's a survival mechanism that prepares the body to either fight or flee from a threat. This response is activated by the sympathetic nervous system and is controlled by hormones, especially adrenaline (epinephrine) and norepinephrine.

**flavonoids** (n.) - A group of plant compounds with antioxidant properties that may protect against disease.

**folate** (n.) - A B-vitamin (B9) naturally found in foods, important for DNA synthesis, cell division, and fetal development.

**follicles** (n.) - Small secretory cavities or sacs, such as those in the skin where hair grows.

**fortified** (adj.) - (Of food) having added nutrients that were not originally present or were lost during processing.

**free radical** (n.) - An unstable molecule with an unpaired electron that can cause cell damage by reacting with other molecules.

**freedom** (n.) - ease of movement or action; absence of barriers.

**frequency** (n.) – 1. rate of occurrence 2. In sound, frequency refers to the number of times a sound wave repeats (or cycles) in one second. It's measured in hertz (Hz). One hertz equals one cycle per second.

**fructose** (n.) - A simple sugar found naturally in fruits, honey, and some vegetables.

**fruition** (n.) – realization; actuality.

**fucoidan** (n.) - A complex sulfated polysaccharide found mainly in brown seaweed, believed to have anti-inflammatory, antiviral, and anticancer properties.

**fucoxanthin** (n.) - A natural pigment (carotenoid) found in brown seaweed and microalgae, known for its antioxidant and potential fat-burning effects.

**functional medicine** (n.) - A holistic approach to healthcare that focuses on identifying and addressing the root causes of disease rather than just treating symptoms.

**fungi** (n.) - A kingdom of spore-producing organisms that includes molds, yeast, mushrooms, and toadstools.

**GABA (Gamma-Aminobutyric Acid)** (n.) - A neurotransmitter in the brain that has a calming effect by inhibiting nerve transmission.

**gastritis** (n.) - Inflammation of the stomach lining, often caused by infection, stress, alcohol, or certain medications.

**genistein** (n.) - A type of isoflavone (plant compound) found mainly in soy products, known for its antioxidant and estrogen-like effects.

**glucose** (n.) - is a type of sugar that your body uses as its main source of energy.

**glucosinolates** (n.) - Naturally occurring sulfur-containing compounds found in cruciferous vegetables like broccoli, kale, and Brussel sprouts.

**glutamic acid** (n.) - A non-essential amino acid involved in cellular metabolism and brain function.

**glutathione** (n.) - A powerful antioxidant naturally produced in the body that helps protect cells from oxidative stress and supports detoxification.

**gluten-free** (adj.) - Describes food or products that do not contain gluten, a protein found in wheat, barley, and rye.

**glycemic index (GI)** (n.) - A system that ranks foods based on how quickly they raise blood sugar levels.

**good cholesterol** (HDL) High-Density Lipoprotein (n.) - known as "good" cholesterol because it helps remove excess cholesterol from the bloodstream.

**govern** (v.) – to hold in check: control.

**grating** (v.) - to scrape or rub with rough or noisy friction, as one thing on or against another.

**grim** (adj.) - Depressing or worrying to consider; bleak.

**gut** (n.) - The digestive tract, especially the intestines.

**gut-brain axis** (n.) - The bidirectional communication network between the gastrointestinal tract and the brain.

**Hawthorn** (n.) - A plant belonging to the Crataegus genus, traditionally used in herbal medicine to support heart health.

**HDL (High-Density Lipoprotein)** (n.) - Known as "good" cholesterol, HDL helps remove excess cholesterol from the bloodstream and transport it to the liver for excretion.

**Healthy fats** (n.) - Types of fats that support health, particularly heart and brain function, such as monounsaturated and polyunsaturated fats. Include omega-3 and omega-6 fatty acids, which can reduce inflammation and support cell health.

**heartburn** (n.) - A burning sensation in the chest caused by acid reflux, where stomach acid backs up into the esophagus.

**hemoglobin** (n.) - A protein in red blood cells that carries oxygen from the lungs to the body's tissues and returns carbon dioxide back to the lungs.

**hertz** (n.) - is the unit of frequency in the International System of Units (SI). It measures how many times an event occurs per second. It is commonly used to describe sound frequencies.

**high-glycemic** (adj.) - Describes foods that cause a rapid spike in blood glucose levels after consumption.

**histamine** (n.) - A chemical compound released by the immune system during allergic reactions, causing symptoms like itching, swelling, and mucus production.

**homeopathic** (adj.) - Relating to homeopathy, a system of alternative medicine based on the principle of treating "like with like" using highly diluted substances.

**homeostasis** (n.) - is the process by which your body maintains a stable internal environment despite changes in the external environment. It ensures that things like body temperature, pH, blood sugar, fluid levels, and blood pressure stay within a healthy range, allowing your cells and organs to function properly.

**hormone** (n.) - a chemical messenger made by glands in your body that travels through your bloodstream to organs and tissues, where it regulates various functions.

**host** (n.) - An organism that harbors a parasite, virus, or another organism (such as gut bacteria), often providing nourishment or shelter.

**(HPA) (Hypothalamic-Pituitary-Adrenal Axis)** (n.) - A complex network involving the hypothalamus, pituitary gland, and adrenal glands that regulates stress response, mood, digestion, immune function, and energy usage.

**hydration (n.) - r**efers to the process of maintaining the balance of fluids in your body. It's the act of ensuring that your body has enough water to perform essential functions and stay healthy.

**Hydrogen** (n.) - is the lightest and most abundant chemical element in the universe. It has the chemical symbol H and an atomic number of 1, meaning it has one proton and usually one electron.

**hydrolyzed protein** (n.) - Protein that has been broken down into smaller peptides or amino acids through a process called hydrolysis, making it easier to digest.

**hygiene** (n.) - Practices that promote health and prevent disease, especially through cleanliness.

**hypertension** (n.) - A medical condition characterized by consistently high blood pressure, increasing the risk of heart disease, stroke, and kidney problems.

**hypothalamus** (n.) - A small region of the brain that controls many bodily functions, including hunger, thirst, temperature regulation, sleep, and hormone release through the pituitary gland.

**IBS (Irritable Bowel Syndrome)** (n.) - A chronic gastrointestinal disorder characterized by abdominal pain, bloating, gas, and changes in bowel habits such as diarrhea or constipation.

**immune function** (n.) - refers to how well your immune system defends your body against infections, diseases, and harmful substances like bacteria, viruses, and toxins. It's your body's natural defense system, made up of cells, tissues, and organs that work together to protect you.

**immune system (n.) -** is your body's defense network made up of cells, tissues, and organs that work together to protect you from harmful invaders like bacteria, viruses, fungi, parasites, and even cancer cells.

**inadequate** (adj.) - Not sufficient or enough in quantity, quality, or degree.

**indigestion** (n.) - Discomfort or pain in the stomach associated with difficulty in digesting food, often experienced as bloating, gas, or a burning sensation.

**Inflammation** (n.) - The body's natural response to injury or infection, characterized by redness, heat, swelling, pain, and sometimes loss of function.

**ingest** (v.) - to take, as food, into the body.

**insidious** (adj.) - Proceeding in a gradual, subtle way but with harmful effects.

**insoluble** (adj.) - Not able to be dissolved in a liquid, especially water.

**insomnia** (n.) - A sleep disorder in which a person has difficulty falling asleep, staying asleep, or getting restful sleep.

**insouciance** (n.) – The act of being free from concern, worry, or anxiety.

**insulin (n.) -** is a hormone made by the pancreas that plays a crucial role in regulating your blood sugar (glucose) levels.

**insulin sensitivity** (n.) - The degree to which the body's cells respond to the hormone insulin, which allows cells to absorb glucose from the bloodstream.

**integrity** (n.) - The state of being whole and undivided; structural soundness.

**intention** (n.) – meaning or significance.

**intestines** (n.) - The long, tube-like organs in the digestive system that absorb nutrients and water from food and remove waste.

**intuition** (n.) - pure, untaught, knowledge.

**invincible** (adj.) - incapable of being conquered, defeated, or subdued.

**iodine (n.) -** A chemical element essential for thyroid function and hormone production.

**Irish Sea Moss** (n.) - is a type of red algae or seaweed that grows along the rocky Atlantic coasts of Europe and North America, especially around Ireland—hence the name. It supports thyroid function, respiratory health, and immune system strength.

**iron** (n.) - A mineral necessary for making hemoglobin, a protein in red blood cells that carries oxygen.

**irregularity** (n.) – The quality or state of not conforming to established rules, customs, etiquette, morality, etc.

**isoflavones** (n.) - Plant-based compounds (phytoestrogens) found in soy and other legumes that may mimic estrogen in the body and provide antioxidant effects.

**jacked up** (adj.) – (slang) messed up

**justification** (n.) - a reason, fact, circumstance, or explanation that defends.

**kaempferol** (n.) - A natural flavonoid (type of antioxidant) found in many fruits and vegetables, known for anti-inflammatory and anti-cancer properties.

**laboratory** (n.) - any place, situation, set of conditions, or the like, conducive to experimentation, investigation, observation, etc.; anything suggestive of a scientific laboratory.

**LDL (Low-Density Lipoprotein)** (n.) - Often referred to as "bad" cholesterol; a type of lipoprotein that transports cholesterol in the blood and can lead to plaque buildup in arteries.

**leaky gut** (n.) - A term used to describe increased intestinal permeability, where the lining of the gut allows undigested food particles, toxins, or bacteria to pass into the bloodstream, potentially triggering inflammation, or immune responses.

**Lecithin** (n.) - A fatty substance found in animal and plant tissues that is essential for cell structure and fat metabolism. It is often used as an emulsifier in foods.

**libido** (n.) - sexual instinct or sexual drive.

**lignans** (n.) - Plant compounds found in seeds (especially flaxseeds), whole grains, and vegetables that have antioxidant and estrogen-like properties.

**linoleic acid** (n.) - An essential omega-6 fatty acid found in many vegetable oils that plays a role in skin health and cellular function.

**lipid** (n.) - A broad group of naturally occurring molecules that include fats, oils, waxes, and cholesterol, important for energy storage and cell membrane structure.

**lipid profiles** (n.) - A blood test that measures levels of specific lipids in the bloodstream, including total cholesterol, LDL, HDL, and triglycerides, to assess cardiovascular risk.

**lot** (n.) - a distinct portion or parcel of anything.

**Low Glycemic Level** (n.) – means it causes a slower, more gradual rise in blood sugar levels.

**Lutein** (n.) - A yellow antioxidant carotenoid found in leafy greens and other vegetables that is important for eye health, particularly in protecting the retina from blue light.

**Lyme** (n.) - Short for Lyme disease, a bacterial infection caused by the *Borrelia* bacterium transmitted through the bite of infected ticks.

**Lymphatic Drainage** (n.) - A therapeutic technique or natural body process that helps move lymph fluid through the lymphatic system to reduce swelling, remove toxins, and support immunity.

**lymphatic system** (n.) - A network of tissues and organs (including lymph nodes, lymph vessels, and lymph fluid) that helps the body remove waste and toxins and plays a key role in immune defense.

**macular degeneration (AMD)** (n.) - A chronic eye disease, particularly in older adults, that causes loss of central vision due to damage to the macula (part of the retina).

**Magnesium** (n.) - An essential mineral involved in over 300 biochemical reactions in the body, including muscle and nerve function, energy production, and bone health.

**Magnesium Glycinate** (n.) - A form of magnesium supplement in which magnesium is bound to the amino acid glycine, known for high absorption and gentle effects on the stomach. Often used for anxiety, sleep, and muscle support.

**manganese** (n.) - A trace mineral essential for bone formation, metabolism, and antioxidant function.

**manifestation** (n.) – A sign or symptom of a condition.

**maturation** (n.) - the process of becoming mature, fully aged or developed, etc.

**melatonin** (n.) - A hormone produced by the pineal gland in the brain that regulates sleep-wake cycles (circadian rhythms).

**menopause** (n.) - The natural biological process marking the end of a woman's menstrual cycles, diagnosed after 12 months without a period, usually occurring between the ages of 45–55.

**metabolic** (adj.) - Related to metabolism—the chemical processes in the body that convert food into energy and maintain life.

**metabolism** (n.) - is the set of chemical processes that occur in your body to convert food into energy and keep you alive and functioning.

**mg/dl** (n.) - It's a unit of measurement used in medical tests to express the concentration of a substance in your blood, especially glucose (blood sugar). mg = milligrams (1/1000th of a gram), dL = deciliter (1/10th of a liter), mg/dL means: how many milligrams of a substance are in one-tenth of a liter of blood.

**microbiome** (n.) - The community of trillions of microorganisms (bacteria, viruses, fungi) that live in and on the human body, especially in the gut, and play a vital role in health and disease.

**micronutrients** (n.) - Essential vitamins and minerals that the body needs in small amounts to function properly.

**migraines** (n.) - A type of recurrent, often severe headache that may include nausea, sensitivity to light or sound, and visual disturbances (auras).

**Minerals** (dietary) (n.) are essential nutrients that your body needs in small amounts to function properly. They come from the foods you eat and help with everything from building bones to maintaining heart rhythm and making hormones.

| Mineral | Main Functions | Common Sources |
|---|---|---|
| Calcium | Bone health, muscle function, nerve signaling | Dairy, leafy greens, fortified foods |
| Magnesium | Muscle/nerve function, energy production | Nuts, seeds, whole grains, leafy greens |
| Potassium | Heart function, fluid balance, muscle control | Bananas, potatoes, beans |
| Sodium | Fluid balance, nerve/muscle function | Table salt, processed foods |
| Phosphorus | Bone formation, energy production | Meat, dairy, nuts |
| Chloride | Works with sodium to maintain fluid balance | Salt, seaweed, vegetables |
| Sulfur | Part of proteins and enzymes | Garlic, onions, eggs, meats |

## 2. Trace Minerals (needed in tiny amounts)

| Mineral | Main Functions | Common Sources |
|---|---|---|
| Iron | Oxygen transport in blood (hemoglobin) | Red meat, spinach, legumes |
| Zinc | Immune support, wound healing | Meat, dairy, nuts |
| Copper | Iron metabolism, nervous system | Shellfish, nuts, seeds |

| Iodine | Thyroid hormone production | Iodized salt, seaweed, dairy |
|---|---|---|
| Selenium | Antioxidant, supports metabolism | Brazil nuts, fish, grains |
| Manganese | Bone health, metabolism | Whole grains, nuts, leafy greens |
| Chromium | Helps regulate blood sugar | Whole grains, broccoli, meat |
| Fluoride | Dental health (strengthens enamel) | Water (in some areas), tea, seafood |
| Molybdenum | Helps enzymes function | Legumes, grains, nuts |

**mineralization** (n.) - The process by which minerals are deposited in body tissues, especially bones and teeth.

**moderation** (n.) - The avoidance of excess or extremes; practicing balance or restraint.

**molecular** (adj.) - Relating to or consisting of molecules, the smallest units of chemical compounds.

**monounsaturated** (adj.) - Describes a type of fat with one double bond in its fatty acid chain, considered heart-healthy. Found in foods like olive oil, avocados, and nuts.

**moral** (n.) - the teaching or practical lesson contained in a fable, tale, experience, etc.

**Most High** (n.) - A title often used to refer to God or a supreme divine being, especially in religious or spiritual contexts.

**mRNA (messenger RNA)** (n.) - A type of RNA that carries genetic information from DNA to the ribosomes, where proteins are synthesized.

**MSG (Monosodium Glutamate)** (n.) - A flavor enhancer commonly added to foods, especially in Asian cuisine and processed products. It is a sodium salt of glutamic acid.

**MSG Symptom Complex (n.) -**

- Headache
- Flushing
- Sweating
- Facial pressure or tightness
- Numbness or tingling
- Chest pain
- Nausea
- Weakness

*These symptoms usually go away on their own and are not considered dangerous.*

**muster** (v.) – to come together, collect, assemble; gather.

**Naan** (n.) - A type of soft, leavened flatbread traditionally baked in a tandoor (clay oven), popular in Indian, Middle Eastern, and Central Asian cuisines.

**Natural Health Improvement Center (NHIC)** is a network of holistic wellness clinics across the United States, dedicated to providing safe, natural solutions for various health concerns. These centers focus on identifying and addressing the root causes of health issues through non-invasive, personalized treatments. (708) 636-5555 www.naturalhealthalsip.com

**negative ion** (n.) - is an atom or molecule that has gained one or more electrons, giving it a net negative electrical charge. They are found abundantly in clean environments like forests, waterfalls, oceans, and after thunderstorms.

**negligence** (n.) – instant of being characterized by paying no attention or too little attention to, disregard.

**neurodegeneration** (n.) - The progressive loss of structure or function of neurons, often associated with diseases like Alzheimer's or Parkinson's.

**neuroendocrine** (adj.) - Relating to interactions between the nervous system and the endocrine system, especially cells that release hormones in response to nerve signals.

**neuroinflammation** (n.) - Inflammation of the nervous tissue, especially in the brain or spinal cord, often associated with neurodegenerative diseases, infections, or trauma.

**neurological** (adj.) - of or relating to the nervous system.

**neurology** (n.) - The branch of medicine that deals with the anatomy, functions, and disorders of the nervous system.

**neuronal** (adj.) - Relating to neurons (nerve cells), which are the primary functional units of the nervous system.

**neurotransmitter** (n.) - is a chemical messenger that carries signals between nerve cells (neurons) in the brain and throughout the nervous system.

**neutralize** (v..) - To counteract or cancel the effect of something. To render something ineffective or harmless.

**neurotransmitter** (n.) - A chemical substance that transmits signals from one neuron to another across a synapse. Examples include serotonin, dopamine, and acetylcholine.

**neurotransmitter synthesis** (n.) - The biological process by which neurons produce neurotransmitters—chemical messengers that transmit signals across synapses.

**Neurotrophin PMG** (n.) - A dietary supplement marketed by Standard Process, claimed to support nervous system health through bovine-derived protomorphogen extracts.

**newfound** (adj.) – newly discovered

**niacin** (n.) - Also known as vitamin B3, niacin is an essential nutrient involved in energy metabolism, DNA repair, and lowering cholesterol levels.

**nitrates** (n.) - Naturally occurring compounds ($NO_3^-$) found in soil, water, and certain vegetables. In the body, nitrates can convert into nitric oxide, which helps relax blood vessels.

**nitrogen (n.)** - a colorless, odorless, gaseous element that constitutes about four-fifths of the volume of the atmosphere and is present in combined form in animal and vegetable tissues, especially in proteins.

**non-heme iron** (n.) - The form of iron found in plant-based foods and fortified products, less easily absorbed by the body compared to heme iron (from animal sources).

**noradrenaline** (n.) - also known as norepinephrine, is both a hormone and a neurotransmitter that plays a central role in the body's stress response, especially the "fight-or-flight" mechanism. It is produced primarily by the adrenal medulla and also released by nerve endings in the sympathetic nervous system.

**norepinephrine** (n.) - A neurotransmitter and hormone involved in the body's "fight-or-flight" response, affecting heart rate, alertness, and blood pressure. Also known as noradrenaline.

**nourishes** (v..) - Provides substances necessary for growth, health, or good condition.

**nutriment** (n.) - anything that nourishes; nourishment; food.

**Nutritional Yeast** (n.) - A deactivated yeast (usually *Saccharomyces cerevisiae*) used as a food product, known for its cheesy, umami flavor and high vitamin B12 content.

**Nutritionist** (n.) - a person who is trained or an expert in the science of the process of nourishing or of being nourished and using food for life, health, and growth.

**observation** (n.) – something that is learned while observing things.

**oleic acid** (n.) - A heart-healthy monounsaturated fatty acid found in olive oil, avocados, and nuts, known for reducing inflammation and supporting cardiovascular health.

**oleocanthal** (n.) - A natural compound found in extra virgin olive oil with anti-inflammatory and antioxidant properties.

**oleuropein** (n.) - A polyphenol found in olive leaves and green olives, known for its antioxidant, anti-inflammatory, and antimicrobial properties.

**olive tapenade** (n.) - A savory spread or dip made from finely chopped or pureed olives, capers, anchovies, and olive oil, common in Mediterranean cuisine.

**omega-3 fatty acids** (n.) - Essential polyunsaturated fats that play a critical role in brain function, heart health, and reducing inflammation. Found in fish (like salmon), flaxseeds, and walnuts.

**omega-6 fatty acids** (n.) - A type of essential polyunsaturated fat important for normal growth and development, but excessive intake (especially in processed foods) may contribute to inflammation.

**onset** (n.) a beginning or start.

**optimal** (adj.) - Best or most favorable; most efficient or effective under specific conditions.

**organic compound** (n.) - are chemical compounds that contain carbon, usually bonded with elements like hydrogen, oxygen, nitrogen, and sometimes sulfur or phosphorus. They are the basis of all life on Earth. They are typically found in living organisms.

**osteoporosis** (n.) - A medical condition in which bones become weak and brittle due to loss of bone density, increasing the risk of fractures.

**overutilize** (v..) – to put to use more than usual

**overwhelmed** (adj.) - Feeling a strong emotional burden, often from stress, anxiety, or responsibility.

**oxidation** (n.) - A chemical reaction in which a substance loses electrons, often producing energy or causing degradation (like rust or rancidity). In the body, it can produce free radicals.

**oxidative stress** (n.) - A harmful condition that occurs when there is an imbalance between free radicals and antioxidants in the body, leading to cell and tissue damage.

**Oxygen** (n.) - a colorless, odorless, gaseous element constituting about one-fifth of the volume of the atmosphere and present in a combined state in nature.

**pantothenic acid** (n.) - Also known as vitamin B5, a water-soluble vitamin essential for synthesizing coenzyme A, which is involved in fatty acid metabolism and energy production.

**parameters** (n.) – limits or boundaries.

**parasite** (n.) - an organism that lives on or in an organism of another species, known as the host, from the body of which it obtains nutriment.

**Parkinson's disease** (n.) is a chronic, progressive neurological disorder that primarily affects movement, caused by the loss of dopamine-producing cells in a part of the brain called the substantia nigra.

**pathogens** (n.) - Microorganisms such as bacteria, viruses, fungi, or parasites that can cause disease.

**pectin (n.)** - A type of soluble fiber found in fruits (especially apples and citrus), used as a gelling agent in food and for promoting digestive health.

**pH** (n.) - is a measure of how acidic or basic (alkaline) a substance is, on a scale from 0 to 14. It reflects the concentration of hydrogen ions ($H^+$) in a solution.

**phenolic compounds** (n.) - A diverse group of chemical substances found in plants, known for their antioxidant properties and health benefits.

**phosphatidylcholine** (n.) - A phospholipid found in cell membranes and a key component of lecithin, important for liver function, brain health, and fat metabolism.

**phosphorus** (n.) - A mineral essential for building bones and teeth, producing energy, and forming DNA and cell membranes.

**phthalides** (n.) - Natural compounds found in certain plants, especially celery, known for their potential to support heart health by relaxing blood vessels and lowering blood pressure.

**phytic acid** (n.) - A natural substance found in seeds, grains, and legumes that stores phosphorus and can bind to minerals like iron and zinc, reducing their absorption in the body.

**phytochemicals (n.)** - Bioactive compounds produced by plants that contribute to color, flavor, and disease resistance, often providing health benefits when consumed.

**phytoestrogens (n.)** - plant-based compounds that mimic the effects of estrogen in the body.

**phytonutrients** (n.) - it's a nutrient that comes from plants and has benefits for human health.

**pigment** (n.) - A natural substance that gives color to plant or animal tissue.

**pigmentation** (n.) - The coloring of an organism's tissues, especially the skin, due to the presence of pigment.

**plane** (n.) - a flat or level surface.

**plaque** (n.) - A fatty deposit inside arteries that contributes to atherosclerosis and cardiovascular disease.

**polyphenolic** (adj.) - Relating to or containing polyphenols; often used to describe plant-based substances with antioxidant properties.

**polyphenols** (n.) - A group of naturally occurring compounds in plants that act as antioxidants and may reduce inflammation and the risk of chronic diseases.

**polyunsaturated fats** (n.) - Healthy fats found in plant and animal foods such as fish, nuts, and vegetable oils. They include omega-3 and omega-6 fatty acids and can help reduce cholesterol levels.

**postmenopausal** (adj.) - Relating to the period in a woman's life after menopause has occurred (when menstrual cycles have permanently stopped).

**potassium** (n.) - helps regulate the balance of fluids inside and outside of cells, ensuring they function properly. It's vital for maintaining a healthy cellular environment. Potassium helps counteract the effects of sodium, which can raise blood pressure.

**potassium chloride** (n.) - A chemical compound used as a potassium supplement or salt substitute; it helps regulate heart function, muscle contraction, and nerve signals.

**prebiotics** (n.) - Types of dietary fiber that feed the beneficial bacteria (probiotics) in the gut, promoting digestive health and overall well-being.

**prediabetes** (n.) - A health condition where blood sugar levels are higher than normal but not high enough to be classified as type 2 diabetes.

**prescribed** (v..) - To have officially recommended or ordered (a medicine or treatment) by a healthcare professional.

**preservative** (n.) - A substance added to food or other products to prevent spoilage, bacterial growth, or chemical change.

**probiotics (n.)** - Live microorganisms (usually bacteria or yeast) that, when consumed in adequate amounts, confer health benefits, especially for the digestive system.

**process** (n.) – A continuous action, operation, or series of changes taking place in a definite manner.

**processed** (adj.) - Refers to food or materials that have been altered from their natural state for safety, convenience, or preservation.

**pronounced** (adj.) – strongly marked.

**protein** (n.) - A macronutrient made of amino acids, essential for building and repairing tissues, enzymes, hormones, and other body chemicals.

**protocols** (n.) - Plans or methods used in clinical or therapeutic settings.

**proton** (n.) - A subatomic particle found in the nucleus of an atom, with a positive electric charge.

**protruding** (adj.) - Sticking out from a surface.

**psycho** (adj.) - crazy; mentally unstable.

**psychological** (adj.) - Relating to the mind or mental processes, especially in regard to behavior or mental health.

**purpose** (n.) - the reason for which something exists or is done, made, used, etc.

**quell (n.)** - to suppress; put an end to; extinguish:

**quercetin** (n.) - A plant pigment (flavonoid) with antioxidant and anti-inflammatory effects, found in foods like onions, apples, and berries.

**quinoa** (n.) - A grain-like seed rich in protein, fiber, and essential amino acids, often used as a healthy substitute for rice or grains.

**rationalize** (v..) - to credit causes that superficially seem reasonable and valid but that actually are unrelated to the true, less creditable causes.

**rear (v.)** - to lift or hold up.

**recollection** (n.) - the act or power of recalling to mind.

**red blood cell** (n.) - A type of blood cell that carries oxygen from the lungs to the body's tissues and returns carbon dioxide from the tissues back to the lungs.

**regimen** (n.) - A systematic plan or course of action, especially one designed to improve or maintain health (e.g., diet, exercise, or medical treatment).

**regularity** (n.) - In health contexts, often refers to consistent bowel movements or bodily functions.

**regulate** (v..) - to adjust to some standard or requirement, as amount, degree, etc.

**rehabilitate (v..)** - to restore to a condition of good health, ability to work, or the like.

**rekindle** (v..) – excite, stir up.

**replenishing** (v..) - Restoring or refilling something that has been used up.

**replete** (adj.) - Fully or abundantly supplied or filled.

**reserpine** (n.) - A medication derived from the Rauwolfia plant, used to treat high blood pressure and certain mental health conditions by affecting neurotransmitters.

**resilience** (n.) - In biology or health, the body's capacity to return to a balanced state after disturbance.

**resistant starch** (n.) - A type of starch that resists digestion in the small intestine and ferments in the large intestine, acting as a prebiotic and supporting gut health.

**respiratory** (adj.) - Relating to the process of breathing or the organs involved in breathing, such as the lungs.

**responsibility** (n.) - the state or fact of being answerable, or accountable for something within one's power, control, or management.

**retina** (n.) - A thin layer of tissue at the back of the eye that detects light and sends visual signals to the brain via the optic nerve.

**Rhodiola** (n.) - A medicinal herb (Rhodiola rosea) used as an adaptogen to help the body resist physical, emotional, and environmental stress.

**Ribonucleic Acid (RNA)** (n.) - A molecule that plays a central role in the coding, decoding, regulation, and expression of genes. RNA carries genetic instructions from DNA to make proteins.

**ribosomes** (n.) - Small cellular structures where proteins are made, using instructions carried by RNA.

**RNA** (n.) - *(Abbreviation for Ribonucleic Acid)* – See definition under **Ribonucleic Acid (RNA)**.

**RNA interference (RNAi)** (n.) - A biological process in which RNA molecules inhibit gene expression or translation, effectively silencing targeted genes.

**sanity** (n.) – the state of being free from mental derangement; having a sound, healthy mind.

**saponins** (n.) - Naturally occurring compounds found in various plants, known for their soap-like foaming properties and potential health benefits like lowering cholesterol and boosting immunity.

**satiety** (n.) - The feeling or state of being full or satisfied, especially after eating.

**saturated fat** (n.) - A type of fat in which all carbon atoms are saturated with hydrogen atoms; found mainly in animal products and some plant oils. Excessive intake may raise cholesterol levels.

**savory** (adj.) - Having a salty or spicy flavor, not sweet.

**Scientologist** (n.) – One who betters the conditions of himself and the conditions of others by using Scientology technology.

**Scientology** (n.) – The science of Knowledge. It is used to increase spiritual freedom, intelligence, and ability, and to produce immortality.

**sedative** (adj.) - Having a calming or tranquilizing effect.

**seizure** (n.) – a sudden attack, as of epilepsy or some other disease.

**Selenium** (n.) - A trace mineral essential for antioxidant defense, thyroid function, and immune health.

**self-deception** (n.) – the act of misleading oneself by false appearance

**serotonin** (n.) - A neurotransmitter involved in mood regulation, appetite, sleep, and digestion. Often referred to as the "feel-good" chemical.

**sesamin** (n.) - A lignan compound found in sesame seeds, known for its antioxidant, anti-inflammatory, and cholesterol-lowering properties.

**sesamol** (n.) - A natural antioxidant compound found in sesame oil, known for protecting cells from oxidative damage.

**severity** (n.) - The condition or quality of being severe, intense, or harsh.

**SIBO (Small Intestinal Bacterial Overgrowth)** (n.) - A condition in which excessive bacteria grow in the small intestine, leading to digestive symptoms like bloating, gas, diarrhea, or malnutrition.

**sodium** (n.) - A mineral and electrolyte essential for maintaining fluid balance, nerve function, and muscle contractions.

**solitude** (n.) - is the state of being alone, often by choice, and not feeling lonely — rather, finding peace, reflection, or clarity in that aloneness.

**soluble** (adj.) - Able to dissolve in a liquid, especially water.

**spasms (n.)** - Sudden, involuntary muscle contractions that may be painful.

**specificity** (n.) – the quality or state of being precise.

**spikes** (n.) - Sharp increases or surges, often in levels such as blood sugar, temperature, or price.

**sprouted tofu** (n.) - A type of tofu made from sprouted soybeans rather than regular soybeans, which may offer enhanced digestibility and increased nutrient availability.

**stability** (n.) – firmness in position.

**stabilize** (v..) - To make or become steady, secure, or less likely to change.

**stead** (n.) - the place of a person or thing as occupied by a substitute

**stimulant** (n.) - Anything that excites or raises levels of physiological or nervous activity.

**stimulant** (n.) - A substance that temporarily increases alertness, energy, or physiological activity in the body, especially the central nervous system.

**stress** (n.) - physical, mental, or emotional strain or tension

**stroke** (n.) – a blockage or hemorrhage of a blood vessel leading to the brain, causing inadequate oxygen supply to parts of the body.

**subacute (adj.)** - refers to a condition or state that is medium in intensity or duration, between acute (sudden and severe) and chronic (long-lasting or persistent).

**subdued** (adj.) - quiet; inhibited; controlled

**subside** (v..) - To lessen, diminish, or become less intense (e.g., symptoms, pain, or weather).

**succumb** (v..) - To yield or give in to a force, temptation, or pressure.

**sucrose** (n.) - A common sugar composed of glucose and fructose, naturally found in many plants, and widely used as table sugar.

**suicidal** (adj.) - pertaining to, involving, or suggesting taking one's own life.

**suit** (v..) - To be appropriate or acceptable for a particular person, condition, or purpose.

**suited** (adj.) – fitted; appropriate for or compatible with a particular person, task, occasion, etc.

**sulfated polysaccharide** (n.) - A complex carbohydrate with sulfate groups attached, often derived from seaweeds and known for biological activity such as anti-inflammatory or antiviral effects.

**sulfur** (n.) - A yellow chemical element (symbol: S) essential for protein structure, detoxification, and enzyme activity in the body.

**sunflower lecithin** (n.) - A natural substance extracted from sunflower seeds, used as an emulsifier in food and supplements, and known for its potential benefits to brain and liver health.

**supplement** (n.) - something added to complete a thing, supply a deficiency, or reinforce or extend a whole.

**suppression** (n.) - The act of stopping or reducing something, such as a process, emotion, or symptom.

**sure-fire** (adj.) - Certain to succeed or be effective.

**sustained** (adj.) - Continuing over a period without interruption; prolonged.

**swiss chard** (n.) - A leafy green vegetable related to beets, rich in vitamins A, C, and K, magnesium, and antioxidants.

**sympathetic nervous system (n.)** - The sympathetic nervous system (SNS) is one of the two main divisions of the autonomic nervous system, which controls involuntary body functions like heart rate, breathing, digestion, and blood pressure. The SNS is best known for activating the body's "fight-or-flight" response during times of stress or danger.

**symptoms** (n.) - Physical or mental features indicating a condition or disease.

**synthesis** (n.) - The process of combining elements to form a whole, especially in biological or chemical systems.

**systemic inflammation** (n.) - A chronic, body-wide inflammatory response that can contribute to various diseases, including heart disease, diabetes, and autoimmune disorders.

**tartar** (n.) - A hard deposit that forms on teeth from plaque buildup and can lead to gum disease.

**thyroid** (n.) - A butterfly-shaped gland in the neck that regulates metabolism, energy, and hormonal balance through the production of thyroid hormones.

**tincture** (n.) - A concentrated herbal extract typically made by soaking plant material in alcohol or another solvent.

**tofu** (n.) - A soft food made from coagulated soy milk, high in protein and used as a meat substitute in vegetarian and vegan diets.

**toxins** (n.) - Poisonous substances produced by living organisms (e.g., bacteria, plants, animals), or synthetic chemicals that can cause harm to the body.

**trauma** (n.) - an experience that produces psychological injury or pain.

**traumatic** (adj.) - of, relating to, or produced by an experience that produces psychological injury or pain.

**tremoring** (n.) - The act or state of trembling.

**trigger** (v..) - To cause something to happen or start, especially suddenly.

**triglycerides** (n.) - A type of fat (lipid) found in the blood, used for energy storage. High levels are associated with an increased risk of heart disease.

**tryptophan** (n.) - An essential amino acid that the body uses to produce serotonin and melatonin, affecting mood and sleep.

**Tulsi (also known as Holy Basil)** (n.) - A medicinal herb (Ocimum sanctum) used in Ayurveda for its adaptogenic, antimicrobial, and anti-inflammatory properties.

**turmoil** (n.) - a state of great commotion, confusion, or disturbance.

**unconscious** (adj.) - without awareness, sensation.

**unsaturated fats** (n.) - Healthy dietary fats that are liquid at room temperature and found in foods like olive oil, avocados, and nuts. They help reduce bad cholesterol levels.

**urination** (n.) – elimination of the liquid-to-semisolid waste matter excreted by the kidneys, in humans, being a yellowish, slightly acidic, watery fluid.

**utmost** (adj.) - of the greatest or highest degree, quantity, or the like.

**UV rays** (n.) - Invisible rays from the sun that can damage the skin, eyes, and DNA, contributing to aging and skin cancer.

**vagus nerve** (n.) - The tenth cranial nerve that extends from the brainstem to the abdomen and plays a crucial role in regulating internal organ functions, including digestion, heart rate, and respiratory rate.

**vasodilation** (n.) - The widening of blood vessels, which decreases blood pressure and increases blood flow.

**vegan** (n.) - A person who does not consume or use any animal products.

**versatile** (adj.) - Able to adapt or be adapted to many different functions or activities.

**vestiges** (n.) - are small remaining parts or traces of something that once existed but is now mostly gone.

**viciously** (adv.) – brutally, ferociously.

**virtually** (adv.) - Almost entirely; nearly.

**vitality** (n.) - The state of being strong and active; energy.

**vitamins** (n.) - Vitamins are organic compounds your body needs in small amounts to function properly and stay healthy. Unlike minerals, which are inorganic, vitamins are carbon-based and are usually obtained from food, because your body either can't make them or can't make enough on its own.

**Vitamin B6** (n.) - A water-soluble vitamin important for brain development, immune function, and the metabolism of proteins and carbohydrates.

**Vitamin B12** (n.) - An essential vitamin that supports nerve function, red blood cell formation, and DNA synthesis. It is found primarily in animal products.

**Vitamin D3** (n.) - A form of vitamin D (cholecalciferol) produced in the skin from sunlight exposure and used to support bone health, immune function, and calcium absorption.

**Vitamin E** (n.) - A fat-soluble antioxidant vitamin that helps protect cells from damage and supports immune function and skin health.

**Vitamins K1** (n.) - A form of vitamin K (phylloquinone) primarily found in green leafy vegetables, involved in blood clotting.

**Vitamins K2** (n.) - A form of vitamin K (menaquinone) that supports bone health and cardiovascular function by helping calcium bind to the right areas in the body.

**Warfarin – (n.)** - is a medication that acts as an anticoagulant (blood thinner). It is used to prevent and treat blood clots in blood vessels, which helps reduce the risk of strokes, heart attacks, or other serious conditions caused by clots.

**ward away** (v..) - To prevent or repel something undesirable, such as illness or danger.

**wean** (v..) - to withdraw one's dependency from some object, habit, form of enjoyment, or the like.

**Westerners** (n.) - People from Western countries, especially Europe and North America.

**whey** (n.) - The liquid part of milk that remains after curdling and straining, often used in protein supplements.

**white blood cells** (n.) - Cells of the immune system that help defend the body against infections and foreign substances.

**wholeheartedly** (adv..) - With complete sincerity, enthusiasm, or commitment.

**zeaxanthin** (n.) - A plant-based carotenoid pigment that acts as an antioxidant, particularly important for eye health as it helps protect the retina from harmful light and oxidative damage.

**Zinc** (n.) is an essential mineral that your body needs in small amounts to function properly. It plays a critical role in immune function, wound healing, DNA synthesis, cell growth, and enzyme activity. Your body can't store zinc, so you need to get it regularly through your diet or supplements.

# About the Author

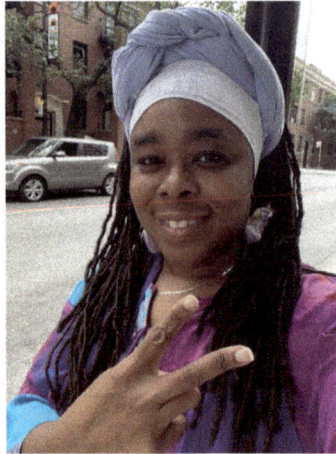

Asadah Kirkland has been meat-free and focused on healthier foods since 1990. She is a multifaceted author, educator, and cultural entrepreneur renowned for her advocacy of positive parenting and the promotion of Black literature. Being born and raised in New York City, Kirkland's early exposure to diverse cultures and experiences shaped her dynamic worldview.

In 2009, Kirkland authored *Beating Black Kids*, a provocative work challenging the normalization of corporal punishment in Black communities. The book advocates for humane parenting practices, aiming to break cycles of generational trauma. Her insights have garnered attention from major media outlets, including CNN and Al Jazeera, and the book has been incorporated into curricula at Old Dominion University.

Recognizing a void in platforms celebrating Black authors, Kirkland founded the Soulful Chicago Book Fair in 2016. This annual event transforms several city blocks into a vibrant literary festival, featuring genres ranging from fiction to children's literature, and includes performances by artists and workshops by authors. In 2022, she expanded the fair into the digital realm with a Metaverse Book Fair, showcasing her adaptability and commitment to innovation.

Beyond her literary endeavors, Kirkland co-authored *Bitcoin for Black People*, aiming to demystify cryptocurrency for African American audiences. Her multifaceted career reflects a dedication to empowering communities through education, literature, and cultural engagement.

www.ingramcontent.com/pod-product-compliance
Lightning Source LLC
Chambersburg PA
CBHW072118020426
42334CB00018B/1642